Facing Hawai'i's Future

Essential Information about GMOs

A project of

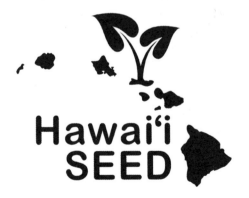

Hawai'i
SEED

Facing Hawai'i's Future (2nd edition)
Essential Information about GMOs
Published by Hawai'i SEED
P.O. Box 1177, Koloa, HI 96756
(808) 652-5286 www.hawaiiseed.org
hawaiiseed@hawaiiseed.org

Compiled by Hawai'i SEED
Edited and designed by Catherine Mariko Black
Front cover art by Solomon Enos
Back cover art by Mayumi Oda

A very special thanks to those who assisted with the preparation of the first edition
of this book, as well as the following individuals: Walter Ritte, Andrew Kimbrell,
Lori Udall, Wailani Artates, Raoul Goff, Mary Lacques, Hector Valenzuela, Cynthia
Franklin, Aiko Yamashiro, Craig Perez and Jeri DiPietro.

Made possible by the Sacharuna Foundation and The Ceres Trust.

ABOUT THE ARTISTS

Solomon Robert Nui Enos is a native Hawaiian artist who was born and
raised on the West side of O'ahu, in Makaha Valley. He is well known for
his celebrated paintings, book illustrations and murals of native Hawaiian
culture and mythology. www.solomonenos.com
Mayumi Oda is a painter and founder of Plutonium Free Future in Japan
and the United States. She lives and farms in Hawai'i. www.mayumioda.net

Printed in China through Palace Press International
ISBN-10: 0615706118
ISBN-13: 978-0-615-70611-5

Table of Contents

La'a Ulu

Na Nancy Redfeather laua'o Kumu Keala Ching

La'a ulu hou a'e	*Spring has returned once again*
Mohala ka ulu	*Renewal of life*
Ulu la'a ulu	*Springs forth*
Ulu a'e nā hua	*From every seed*
Kau pono nā hua	*Seeds of the Ancestors*
Naue mai, naue mai	*Awaken the Ancestors*
Nā iwi o ka 'āina	*Ancestors of the Land*
Īnana nā kupa	*Life stirs within us*
Pili pa'a pono	*Come together*
No ka wailua ala	*Connect with*
Ala pono ka wailua	*The ancient knowledge*
Kau pono nā hua	*Seeds of the Ancestors*
Naue mai, naue mai	*Awaken the Ancestors*
Nā iwi o ka 'āina	*Ancestors of the Land*
Hua a'e ka wailua	*Knowledge of the seed*
Wailua ka hua	*Seed of Life*
Hua hiwa iho ala	*Precious seed of Life*
Ho'ālahia	*Awaken!*
Kau pono nā hua	*Seeds of the Ancestors*
Naue mai, naue mai	*Awaken the Ancestors*
Nā iwi o ka 'āina	*Ancestors of the Land*

A resident of Kealakehe, Kona, Hawai'i, Kumu Keala Ching is a Hawaiian Cultural Educator, composer, song writer and spiritual advisor to many Hawaiian organizations. He is co-founder and Executive Director of Nā Wai Iwi Ola (NWIO) Foundation, which perpetuates Hawaiian culture and practices through hula protocol and ceremonies, the use and study of the Hawaiian language, and by embracing the stories of our kupuna past. Kumu Ching is kumu hula of Ka Pā Hula Nā Wai Iwi Ola and Nā Wai Puna o Kona (Kūpuna) in Kailua-Kona and is a kumu and cultural advisor to a number of hula hālau in Hawai'i, the U.S. mainland and abroad.

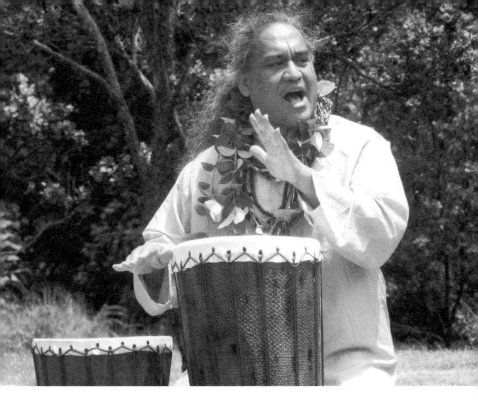

The seeds of knowledge are the seeds of our ancestors. We honor them by knowing them and living their legacy within our everyday life. Moving forward with the knowledge of our ancestors keeps them very near; they are a part of who we are within the world we live in now. Laʻa Ulu recognizes the beauty and the seeds of knowledge that our ancestors have built for us, and it is our responsibility to continue to allow the beauty of this legacy for the future generations to live!

The future is seeded by our actions today. The time has come for the renewal of agriculture. Seeding the future with the wisdom and knowledge of the past combined with the best of the new ecological and sustainable agricultural techniques available today will allow a healthy food and farming future to unfold for our children. It is up to us to care for the land in such a way that it will not be compromised for the future generations to come.

Eō Laʻa Ulu ē!

O Ke Au Mua, O Ke Au Nei

From the knowledge deep within until the knowledge of the present time...

The Hawaiian Islands stand isolated and unique, alone in a vast sea. The complex ecosystems that form life here evolved slowly over eons of geologic time. Hawai'i is a "hotspot" of biodiversity with more species of endangered plants and animals than anywhere else on Earth.

This priceless living treasure, however, is under siege. Development, increasing population and climate change all put pressure on Hawai'i's ecosystems. Alien species, with increasing frequency, overtake our natives, erasing our opportunity to understand the intricate web of life which surrounds us and of which we are part.

Today, we can see an approaching food and farming tsunami. The revolution occurring in agriculture has the potential to forever change the basic genetic structure of the food we eat, as well as the soils, the plants, and the animals that form the delicate balance of our pristine ecosystem. Multinational corporations and universities with the full support of federal and state governments are altering the genetic structure and nutritional content of the foods we eat, patenting the seed, preventing farmers from saving seed, and changing the course of 10,000 years of agriculture. Genes of different species are being combined in food crops at the molecular level without knowledge of their effects on ecosystems or human health.

Years ago, a decision was made to allow Hawai'i to become the nursery for experimental genetically engineered agricultural crops known as GMOs (genetically modified organisms). Big corporations have big influence and our year-round growing season, geographical isolation and permissive regulations each contributed their part. Unfortunately, co-existence of conventional (non-GMO), organic and GMO agriculture is not biologically possible.

There is so much to preserve and protect in our islands, yet GMOs will never give us the truly diversified food production and food security we need. Many people have a different vision of Hawai'i's path to an ecological and sustainable agricultural future. This vision is grounded in recycling the vast bounty of organic materials available in the tropics to produce soil and ecosystem health; in wise choices of planting varieties and growing season; and in a better understanding of the complex interaction between 'āina and culture. Imagine a proud and independent Hawai'i filled with unique varieties of locally produced tropical foods grown on diverse family farms.

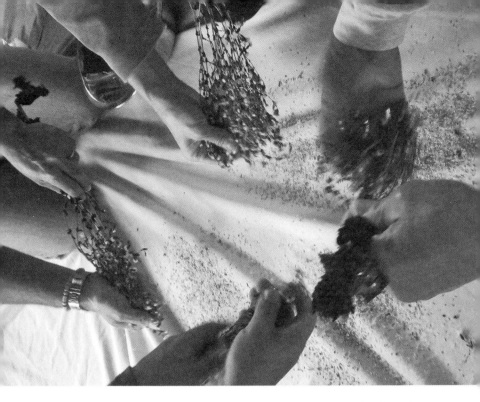

Imagine our islands as a mecca not just for recreation but also for health and wellness, an example to the world. Imagine our state and county agencies and our university system supporting these ideas.

Hawai'i SEED is a grassroots coalition of farmers, consumers, parents, doctors and scientists from every corner of the Hawaiian islands. Now is the time to bring increased awareness and speak openly about GMO agriculture and its effects on the environment, health and culture of Hawai'i's people. We hope to grow a vision for a more sustainable form of agriculture based on statewide support for local, diversified farms and aware, engaged communities. It is not too late for Hawai'i to bring that vision to life.

As you read the stories in this compilation, some frightening and others inspiring, we ask you to keep this vision in mind. This book is meant to be used as a tool for change, an opportunity to build the future that our children and their children deserve. Pale ke ao – protect what is here now.

Hawai'i SEED is a nonprofit organization and coalition of grassroots groups from five islands including GMO-Free Kaua'i, GMO-Free O'ahu and GMO-Free Maui.

What is Genetic Engineering?
Basic Definitions and Concepts

Luke Anderson

Genetic engineering or "GE" is a laboratory technique used to make new kinds of plant, animal or other living organisms. It is now possible, using these techniques, to cross natural boundaries and force together DNA from any different species, such as inserting jellyfish genes in corn plants or human genes in rice. Examples of genetic engineering experiments that have already been done include:

- Spider/Goat – taking a gene from a spider that leads to the production of spider web and putting it into goats so the goats can then be milked for the spider web protein.
- Fish/Strawberries – taking a gene from an Arctic flounder and putting it into a strawberry to try to make it frost-resistant.
- Corn/Human – taking a human gene and putting it into corn so that the corn contains human antibodies that attack sperm. The idea is to develop the corn as a plant-gel contraceptive that kills sperm on contact.

Hawai'i has the highest recorded number of open-air experiments with genetically engineered plants in the world. Examples include:

- Corn engineered with human genes (Dow)
- Sugarcane engineered with human genes (Hawai'i Agriculture Research Center)
- Corn engineered with jellyfish genes (Stanford University)
- Tobacco engineered with lettuce genes (University of Hawai'i)
- Rice engineered with human genes (Applied Phytologics)
- Corn engineered with hepatitis virus genes (Prodigene)[1]

What is a gene?
Every plant and animal is made of cells, each of which has a center called a nucleus. Inside every nucleus there are strings of DNA, half of which is normally inherited from the mother and half from the father. Short sequences

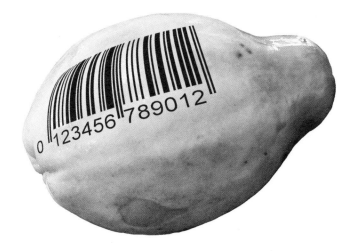

of DNA are called genes. These genes operate in complex networks that are finely regulated to enable the processes of living organisms to occur in the right place and at the right time.

Haven't we been breeding new plants and animals for thousands of years? Isn't that just like genetic engineering?

Genetic engineering is completely different from traditional breeding. In traditional breeding it is possible to mate a pig with another pig to obtain a new breed, but it is not possible to mate a pig with a potato or a mouse. Even when species that may seem to be closely related do succeed in breeding, the offspring are usually infertile – a horse, for example, can mate with a donkey, but the offspring (a mule) is sterile.

How is genetic engineering done?

Because living organisms have natural barriers to protect themselves against the introduction of DNA from a different species, genetic engineers have to find ways to force the DNA from one organism into another. These methods include:

- Using viruses or bacteria to "infect" animal or plant cells with the new DNA.
- Using electric shocks to create holes in the membrane covering sperm, and then forcing the new DNA into the sperm through these holes.
- Injecting the new DNA into fertilized eggs with a very fine needle.
- Coating DNA onto tiny metal pellets, and firing it with a special gene gun into a layer of plant cells.

Is genetic engineering precise?

The technology of genetic engineering is currently very crude. It is not possible to insert a new gene with any accuracy, and the transfer of new genes can disrupt the finely controlled network of DNA in an organism.

Current understanding of the way in which DNA works is extremely limited, and any change to the DNA of an organism at any point can have short or long-term side effects that are impossible to predict or control. The new gene could, for example, alter chemical reactions within the cell or disturb cell functions. This could lead to genetic instability, to the creation of new toxins or allergens, and to changes in nutritional value.

For example, when genetically engineered salmon were compared to normal salmon, it was found that the genetic engineering unexpectedly increased the amount of a protein identified as a major food allergen.[3] In another case, Australian researchers reported that after 10 years spent developing a genetically engineered pea they had to abandon the project after they found out that the altered peas caused lung inflammation and other adverse effects in mice.[4] "The reaction of the mice . . . might reflect something that would happen to humans," said deputy chief of CSIRO plant industry T. J. Higgins.[5]

Why do genetically engineered foods have antibiotic resistant genes in them?

The techniques used to transfer genes have a very low success rate, so the genetic engineers attach "marker genes" that are resistant to antibiotics to help them to find out which cells have taken up the new DNA. These marker genes are resistant to antibiotics that are commonly used in human and veterinary medicine. Some scientists believe that eating GE food containing these marker genes could encourage gut bacteria to develop antibiotic resistance.

The British Medical Association[6] stated in 1999 that, "Antibiotic

GE, GMOs and Biotechnology

Genetic engineering is sometimes called "genetic modification," and a genetically engineered organism is often called a GMO. Another word that is occasionally used to talk about genetic engineering is "biotechnology." This word can be confusing, because "biotechnology" is very general, and includes all the different ways humans work with living organisms, (e.g. using yeasts to make bread or beer). There are many kinds of biotechnology that have nothing to do with the genetic engineering of agriculture or the release of GMOs into the environment.

resistance, the threat of new allergic reactions and the unknown hazards of transgenic DNA mean that on health grounds alone the impact of GMOs must be fully assessed before they are released. The environmental implications and the long term effects on human health cannot be safely predicted at this stage and caution must therefore prevail."

Lorrin Pang, MD, and MPH Advisor to the World Health Organization echoes those concerns relative to Hawai'i's genetically engineered papaya. "The genetically engineered papaya contains three antibiotic resistant marker (ARM) genes. I am concerned about the possibility that they might transfer to the human gut bacteria, and then create new disease strains that will be resistant to the three important antibiotics."

Isn't genetically engineered food safety tested?

The United States regulatory agencies such as the FDA have deregulated GMOs. What this means is that in most cases it is left up to the corporations themselves (those who stand to profit from the introduction of genetically engineered crops) to decide whether or not their products are safe. There is no long-term safety testing of genetically engineered food. The genetic engineering corporations sometimes conduct short-term animal feeding trials, but most of this research is kept confidential. Neither the public, farmers, elected officials nor regulatory agencies are given vital information that would be needed to determine safety concerns associated with these experiments.

No evidence from human trials for either toxicity or allergy testing is required. No independent checks of the company's claims are required. Because GE products in the market are not labeled, the corporations producing GMOs have also avoided liability that would hold them accountable in case of any hazardous effects.

But nobody's fallen over dead from eating genetically engineered food, have they?

Proponents of genetic engineering often make comments such as: "We've been eating GE food for years in the United States and there have been no problems. No one has even caught a cold." Considering that there have been no long-term studies (following people who have eaten GE food over years, comparing them with a group of people who have not eaten GE food, taking blood samples, etc.) how would we know if people are being affected? Many scientists feel that an evaluation of GE food would require studying the cumulative effects of eating it over many years. Because GE products are not labeled, it is also nearly impossible to conduct post-marketing studies to detect any short or long-term health effects on consumers.

"This technology is being promoted, in the face of concerns by respectable scientists and in the face of data to the contrary, by the very agencies which are supposed to be protecting human health and the environment," says Dr. Suzanne Wuerthele, a toxicologist with the U.S. Environmental Protection Agency (EPA). "The bottom line in my view is that we are confronted with the most powerful technology the world has ever known, and it is being rapidly deployed with almost no thought whatsoever to its consequences."

Why isn't genetically engineered food labeled in the United States?

Examples from around the world show that when GE food is labeled, people vote with their wallets and boycott food containing genetically engineered ingredients. The industry has lobbied hard to prevent labeling in the U.S., spending more than $45 million, for example, to defeat Proposition 37, a citizens' labeling initiative on the 2012 California ballot.

The fact that GMO foods are not labeled as such eliminates traceability of these products in the food chain, and does not allow for the tracking of food illnesses and allergic reactions. Countries around the world with labeling of GMOs include Australia and New Zealand, Brazil, China, the Czech Republic, all 15 countries of the European Union, Hong Kong, Israel, Japan, Latvia, Mexico, Norway, the Philippines, Poland, the Republic of Korea, Russia, Saudi Arabia, Switzerland, Taiwan and Thailand.

Don't GMOs reduce the use of pesticides?

A 2003 study which analyzed the U.S. Department of Agriculture's own statistics found that pesticide use actually increased by about 50 million pounds with the planting of genetically engineered crops from 1996-2003.[9] This is hardly surprising – the corporations selling genetically engineered crops own 60 percent of the global pesticide market.[10] These are not corporations that want to see farmers using fewer chemicals; these are corporations that want to profit by selling more of their chemicals.

More than 70 percent of the genetically engineered crops that are grown are crops engineered to be resistant to these corporations' own-brand chemicals.[11] A GE pesticide resistant crop means that a farmer can liberally spray the field with the chemicals without harming the genetically engineered crop. Herbicide-resistant genes are being transferred from genetically engineered crops to weeds via cross-pollination, and higher and higher doses of chemicals are being needed to have the desired effect, leading to a rise in herbicide use.

How can GMOs cause pollution?

Genetically engineered organisms are alive. This means that once they are released into the environment, genetically engineered plants and animals can reproduce and contaminate any other plants or animals with which they can breed. In many cases genetically engineered organisms can never be recalled or contained after they have been released, and any problems could then multiply for future generations. One example is a study at Purdue University, where researchers studied the potential effects of the release of a small number of genetically engineered fish into the wild. They estimated that just 60 genetically engineered fish released into a wild population of 60,000 could lead to the extinction of the wild fish within 40 generations.[12]

"Open-air testing of genetically engineered plants in vulnerable ecosystems presents unacceptable risks to Hawai'i's fragile biodiversity," says Cha Smith, former executive director of KAHEA, an alliance of Hawaiian and environmental activists. "Pollen from plants that are engineered to produce powerful chemicals will assuredly be carried by trade winds and eaten by insects and birds. There is no way to prevent the spread of genetic material to native plants and animals."[13]

Luke Anderson is the author of the book "Genetic Engineering, Food and Our Environment." Since 1997 he has worked with environmental, farming and social justice groups around the world as an advisor on GE-related issues.

Fit for Human Consumption?
Health Effects of Genetically Engineered Food

Elisha Goodman

It is difficult to find independent funding to conduct unbiased health studies of genetically engineered (GE) crops. Studies conducted or funded by GE crop developers may be skewed to their advantage and troubling results may be withheld from summary data shown to regulators and the public. This was the case with Monsanto's insecticide-producing GE corn, called MON863.[1] Summary data from a 90-day rat feeding study revealed to European regulators raised concerns, prompting requests for release of the full study, which had been conducted by Monsanto. The company refused to comply, acceding only a year later upon order of a German court. A reanalysis of the data submitted by Monsanto and reviewed by independent scientists revealed that rats fed MON863 had lower kidney weights and elevated white blood cell counts compared to rats fed conventional corn. Independent reviewers who called for further studies to establish whether the corn posed human health risks were ignored.

The list below contains just a few of the independent studies and their results indicate that we should have grave concern about the health effects of GMOs.

Genes from GMOs Transfer to Bacteria in Humans

Genes engineered into one organism have transferred to bacteria in the mouth[2] and gut of humans.[3] In one of the only human feeding studies ever conducted to test GMOs, it was found that before the trial even began, three out of seven of the subjects' gut bacteria had already experienced gene transfer from genetically modified (GM) soy. The fact that the bacteria took up the Roundup Ready® trait is an example of horizontal gene transfer, a phenomenon long discounted by the biotech industry. Most worrying, these studies show the potential for bacteria to also take up antibiotic resistant genes often engineered into GMOs. Bacteria could then become resistant to the antibiotics we use against diseases and fail to be cured by antibiotics.

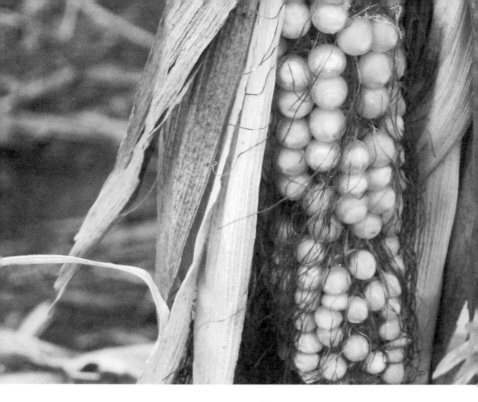

Mice Fed GM Peas Show Immune Response

Mice that were fed peas engineered with a gene from a bean demonstrated an immune response, including inflammation of the lungs and increased serum antibody levels.[4] Significantly, the protein produced from the natural version of the same gene in beans does not cause these responses. The study shows that heedlessly transferring genes from one organism to another via genetic engineering can have health consequences, including allergies and other adverse immune responses.

Allergic Reaction Caused By Gene Engineered into Soy

A gene from the Brazil nut inserted into soybeans made the soy allergenic to those who normally react to Brazil nuts.[5]

GM Soy Contains Proteins Identical to Shrimp and Dust Mite Allergens

Unlike regular soy, the GM soy consumed in the United States contains protein sections that are identical to those found in shrimp and dust mite allergens.[6] This GM soy is the most widely grown GM crop, and in the form of soy formula is often fed to infants, yet there were never follow-up studies done to determine whether the soy is in fact allergenic.

Rats Fed GM Potatoes Have Pre-cancerous Cell Growth and Gastric Problems

A UK government-funded study demonstrated that rats fed GM potatoes developed potentially pre-cancerous cell growth and gastric problems.[7]

GM Corn-Fed Rats Have Problems with Blood Cell, Kidney and Liver Formation

Rats fed Monsanto's GM corn, MON 863, had problems with blood cell, kidney and liver formation.[8] Male rats had increased white blood cells and female rats had lower levels of red blood cells. Livers and kidneys had lesions and malformations.

No Minimum Level of GMO StarLink Corn Judged Safe for Human Consumption

After StarLink contaminated the food supply, expert scientific advisors to the EPA stated that there was no minimal level of StarLink's Cry9C insecticidal protein that could be judged safe for human consumption.[9] An extensive literature review reveals numerous unpublished studies that indicate the insecticidal proteins engineered into Bt corn may be allergenic.[10]

GM Produced Tryptophan Associated With At Least 37 Deaths and 1500 Serious Illnesses

A batch of tryptophan produced by GM microorganisms was associated with at least 37 deaths and 1500 disabilities from a rare disease known as eosinophilia-myalgia syndrome.[11]

Unpredictable Biotech Techniques Could Lead to Toxic Carcinogenic Products

According to Salk Institute cell biologist David Schubert, the crude and unpredictable nature of genetic engineering techniques could lead to "the biosynthesis of molecules that are toxic, allergenic or carcinogenic ... GM food is not a safe option, given our current lack of understanding of the consequences of recombinant technology."[12]

Elisha Goodman has lived and worked on organic farms in Hawai'i and abroad. She is the former director of Hawai'i SEED and sits on the Board of Trustees of the Hawai'i Organic Farmers Association.

Pesticide Use in Crop Biotechnology
Concerns and Calls to Action

Dr. Héctor Valenzuela

Pesticide Use in the United States

Synthetic pesticides became an integral part of conventional agricultural systems since they were first developed and manufactured on an industrial scale during the 1940s and 1950s. Since their introduction early in the last century, farmers continued to increase their reliance on the use of pesticides as a central feature of their pest control programs, for the management of weeds, arthropod pests and diseases. For example, from 1992 to 1997, insecticide use in the United States increased by 18 percent from about 67,000 to over 82,000 tons per year.[1] By 2001, over 400,000 tons of pesticides (active ingredient) were used in the United States, with herbicides representing 64 percent, and insecticides 11 percent of the total use of pesticides.[2] The use of pesticides is extensive with some mainstream crops in the United States. For example over 90 percent of farmers in the United States relied on herbicides to control weeds in corn during the early 1990s,[3] and this level probably increased to close to 100 percent with the introduction of herbicide resistant genetically engineered (GE) corn varieties during the mid-90s.

The increased use of synthetic pesticides occurred hand-in-hand with the industrialization of agricultural systems. This took place in the form of the increased use of large-scale monoculture plantings; mechanization; less use of crop rotations; a consolidation or increase in the size of conventional farms; and an overall vegetational simplification of agricultural landscapes.

Human Health Concerns about the Use of Pesticides

The publication of *Silent Spring* by Rachel Carson in 1962 was among the first popular works that raised warnings and awareness about environmental and health risks from the widespread application of pesticides. Follow-up studies led by Cornell University Professor David Pimentel documented that pesticides pose "serious impacts" on human health and on the environment. He and his colleagues estimated societal costs of $12 billion per year from the negative environmental and human health impacts of the legal use of pesticides in the United States.[4]

The U.S. General Accountability Office, Congress' independent research branch, recognized that pesticides pose considerable "unintended" consequences for health and the environment in its call for a wider adoption of Integrated Pest Management (IPM) practices in the United States. These consequences include "increased risks for cancer, neurological disorders, and endocrine and immune system dysfunction; impaired surface and ground water; and harm to fish and wildlife."[5]

Of the 1,400 pesticides that have been approved by the U.S. Environmental Protection Agency, exposure to some has been linked to several cancers including brain/central nervous system (CNS), breast, colon, lung, ovarian, pancreatic, kidney, testicular and stomach cancers, as well as Hodgkin and non-Hodgkin lymphoma, multiple myeloma and soft tissue sarcoma. Those more directly exposed to pesticides such as applicators or manufacturers have also been found to have higher rates of prostate cancer, melanoma, other skin cancers and cancer of the lip. Overall, according to the President's Cancer Panel, the total number of registered pesticides in the United States that contain known or suspected carcinogens is "far greater than 40."[6]

According to the President's Cancer Panel, registered pesticides overall contain about 900 active ingredients. Many of the inert ingredients used in pesticide formulation are also toxic, but are not required to be tested. Xylene is an example of an inert ingredient that is found in over 900 pesticides, and its exposure to humans has been associated with brain tumors, rectal cancer and leukemia.[7]

Studies have also indicated that exposure to pesticides may affect the respiratory system. A survey of pesticide applicators showed that 15 percent suffered asthma, chronic sinusitis, or chronic bronchitis, compared to only 2 percent for people exposed to pesticides infrequently.[8] More recent research has found evidence that certain synthetic chemicals, referred to as "obesogenes" – including agricultural pesticides such as atrazine, DDE (a breakdown product of DDT), clorpyriphos, diazinon and parathion – may contribute to increased obesity in exposed populations. Research indicates that these chemicals may alter metabolic pathways, predisposing some people to gain weight.[9]

National agricultural policies may also have unintended health impacts on rising obesity trends. A recently released publication on obesity by the National Academy of Sciences indicates that agricultural subsidies of

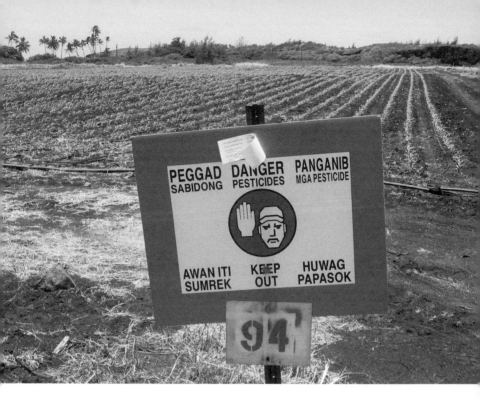

"obesogenic" foods, many of which are produced from subsidized genetically modified crops such as GE corn and GE soybean, may be contributing to the overconsumption of these foods and to the obesity epidemic in the United States.[10] Whether pesticide residues in these subsidized crops are causing further negative health impacts on the population remains to be investigated.

Use of Pesticides in GE Crops

The intensive use of pesticides is an integral part of the first generation of crops that have been produced through genetic engineering. Today over 95 percent of the GE acreage globally consists of either GE varieties that produce pesticides themselves, or that were developed to tolerate overhead applications of herbicides as a central feature of the weed management program. By 2006, over 80 percent of the total acreage planted in GE crops consisted of varieties with an herbicide-tolerant trait, representing over 200 million acres. Similarly, herbicide-resistant Roundup-ready varieties in 2010 represented 90 percent of the soybean, and 80 percent of the corn acreage planted in the United States. Overall, in the United States the use of Roundup (Glyphosate) more than doubled, from 85-90 million pounds in 2001, to over 180 million pounds in 2007.

Since the introduction of GE crops the global use of Roundup (Glyphosate) herbicide has expanded considerably. However as some weeds have developed resistance to Roundup, farmers have begun to apply some of the older herbicides that were used in the past. The use of the Bt pesticide, which was engineered to be produced by the plant itself, has also expanded considerably. As caterpillar pests develop resistance to Bt, growers are increasingly relying on other insecticides, and on multiple pesticide applications, to manage pest populations.

GE growers have also had to rely on the application of conventional pesticides for new pests that are developing, or to manage the outbreak of what were formerly considered minor or secondary pests. This phenomenon was documented with the outbreak of mirid bugs in Bt cotton fields in China[11] and with the increased aphid populations observed in Bt corn compared to non-GE varieties.[12]

Environmental and Health Risks from the Use of Pesticides in GE Crops

Minimal research focus has been given to assess the environmental and health risks from the use of pesticides in crop biotechnology. An assessment on the impact of pesticides used for the production of GE crops should include both pesticides that are used as part of the production program, such as the herbicide Roundup (Glyphosate), as well as any pesticides that have been engineered into the plant, such as the one found in the Bt GE crops (Bacillus thuringiensis).

A recent report from Europe unearthed studies from the refereed research literature and from studies submitted by industry to European regulators, on potential health risks from exposure to the herbicide Roundup (Glyphosate). Adverse health effects reported from this European study include birth defects; death of the fetus; lung, kidney, heart and skeletal malformations; endocrine disruption; damage to liver cells; human cell death; DNA damage or genotoxic effects; cancer; and neurotoxic or nervous system effects.[13] Recently researchers from France reported on the first-ever long-term study on the effect of Roundup on mice. While most animal studies on the health impacts of Roundup conducted to date have lasted only 90 days, this study was conducted over two years, covering the entire life-span of the laboratory animals. Adverse health impacts from this first refereed long-term study on the exposure of Roundup included tumor development, cancer, organ damage and early death, compared to control animals receiving a non-GE diet.[14]

The number of studies evaluating the environmental impact from the use of pesticides used for the production of GE crops is also limited. With respect to the intensive use of Roundup (Glyphosate) in agricultural systems, research from Argentina showed that its use in pastures had a negative impact on landscape biodiversity.[15] Similarly, in the United States researchers found an 80 to 90 percent reduction in the populations of milkweed in Roundup-treated fields of Iowa. In turn, the reduction of milkweed populations at the landscape level may help to explain the observed reductions in monarch butterfly populations overwintering in Mexico.[16]

Another environmental impact from the extensive use of herbicides for the production of GE crops is the development of "superweeds" or weeds that become resistant to herbicide applications. This creates a problem because the resulting weed biotypes are increasingly difficult to manage on farms or in conservation areas. To date 18 weed species have been found to show resistance to Roundup (Glyphosate) applications.[17] In contrast to the idea that weed control can be centered on the application of one herbicide, weed specialists from Iowa State University now claim that "full-season weed control from one herbicide treatment is a myth devised by ad agencies," and now recommend that farmers instead follow integrated management programs. According to these weed specialists, the production models based on the planting of herbicide resistant GE crops "tend to emphasize simplicity and convenience resulting in the recurrent use of single herbicides."[18]

The extensive use of pesticides in conventional agricultural systems has been mentioned as a possible variable contributing toward the decline of bee populations in many parts of the world. Among the pesticides suspected to have contributed toward bee population declines include the neonicotinoids, which are used for seed treatments in many GE crops.[19]

Another area of human health and environmental concern is the number and quantity of pesticides used for the seed production of GE crops. In Hawai'i for instance it is estimated that over 70 different pesticides are used to grow GE crops for breeding, research and seed production. When dealing with multiple pesticide applications in time and space, concerns apply not only to the individual chemical ingredients, but also their breakdown products, as well as to the interaction between the different chemicals, which could possibly result in more dangerous secondary metabolites or new toxics.[20]

Environmental concerns with respect to the use of pesticides for GE seed production include pesticides reaching non-target organisms, aquifers, aquatic habitats and nearby communities, as well as soil pollution. Examples of pesticides used by the seed industry in Hawai'i that may reach non-target areas include Atrazine, Chlorpyrifos (Lorsban), Prowl (Pendimethalin), and Bacillus thuringiensis (via fugitive dust); atrazine, chlorpyrifos, cyfluthrin, Lambda-cyhalothrin (Warrior), dimethoate, metolachlor, 2,4-D, Dicamba, and Roundup (Glyphosate) (via drift); atrazine, alachlor (Lasso), bromoxynil (Buctril), carbaryl, chlorpyrifos, dimethoate, dicamba (Banvel), Glyphosate (Roundup), Lorsban (chlorpyrifos), metolachlor (Dual), methyl parathion (Penncap-M), nicosulfuron (Accent), Permethrin, and Simazine (Princep), which may be found in aquatic habitats or surface waters.[21]

Pesticides used by the GE seed industry for which adverse health effects have been reported based on animal or epidemiological studies include Atrazine, Lorsban (Chlorpyrifos), Roundup (Glyphosate), 2,4-D, Alachlor (Lasso), Bentazon (Basagran), Carbaryl, Dicamba, Dimethoate, Glufosinate, Metolachlor, Permethrin, simazine (Princep) and Bacillus thuringiensis.[22]

Another environmental concern with the planting of GE crops involves soil nutrient or fertility imbalances in fields that have been treated with Roundup herbicide. Several studies have documented significant Roundup micronutrient interactions in the soil, leading to increased disease susceptibility for either the current crop, or for crops to be grown in the same field in the months or years following the initial Roundup application. The increased incidence of some diseases in crops after soil Roundup applications has been documented for over 15 years.[23]

Calls for Alternative Strategies to Pest Control

By the 1970s many mainstream pest management specialists had realized that, "Rather than solving pest problems, the extensive use of pesticides often has resulted in a combination of new problems without eliminating the old ones" and that "pesticides often are still used without regard to detrimental side effects." According to these scientists, the negative side effects from an overreliance on pesticides included pesticide residues in food, biomagnification (or accumulation of pesticides in the food chain), and the development of resistant and secondary pests.[24]

Because of the concerns about the increased dependence on synthetic chemical inputs, mechanization of agriculture, and potential environmental and health impacts, the U.S. Congress enacted the 1985 Food Security

Act calling for the establishment of a program to research and disseminate information on alternative agricultural systems.[25] To reduce this overreliance on the use of pesticides, the concept of Integrated Pest Management (IPM) was developed in the 1960s and 70s to encourage the adoption of alternative management practices to minimize the use of pesticide applications. In fact, within the IPM approach, pesticide use was considered a "last resort" after all other control options had been exhausted.[26] The IPM approach was thus promoted by mainstream agricultural scientists because, among other things, it could lead to "a substantial reduction in pesticide residues" in food, and also to "an improved environment."[27]

More recently, recommendations for alternative production methods that reduce the reliance on the use of pesticide and intensive industrial production methods were made at the UN Rio Earth Summit of 1992, and in 2008 by the International Assessment of Agricultural Knowledge, Science, and Technology for Development (IAASTD). The IAASTD report was prepared by 400 scientists from about 60 countries, and calls for a greater focus on alternative agroecological approaches.[28]

Today, university extension programs for the production of GE crops are also recommending an increased reliance on alternative pest control methods, especially to deal with emerging problems such as the development of herbicide resistant weeds, which may result from an overreliance on herbicide applications.[29] Similar calls for alternative management strategies have been made to address the growing problem of insect pests developing resistance to GE Bt crops.[30]

Alternative Management Strategies for Pest Control

Agricultural ecologists believe that it is possible to adopt alternative production practices that minimize, or eliminate completely the need for synthetic pesticides. Pesticide reduction practices have already been implemented successfully in several countries and regions. Sweden, Canada and Indonesia have implemented programs to reduce their pesticide use by 50 to 65 percent without sacrificing crop yields nor quality.[31] During the 1980s and early 1990s in the United States, prior to the introduction of GE crops, conventional growers in several states were able to drastically reduce the amount of pesticides used. For instance, in Alabama cotton growers planting over 420,000 acres were able to reduce annual pesticide applications by 40 percent. In California, almond growers planting in over 430,000 acres were able to reduce insecticide applications by 78 percent without reducing yields or quality. And in Texas, cotton growers were able to reduce pesticide applications by nearly 88 percent, by adopting IPM, over a 10-year period.[32] Since the 1960s biologists, agricultural scientists and policy makers have warned about the environmental and human health implications of an overreliance on pesticides as a central feature of pest control programs. During the 1970s IPM programs were developed in which pesticide use was relegated as a tool of "last resort." During the 1990s with the introduction of GE crops, pesticides once again became a central and prominent feature of modern agricultural systems. Over the first 13 years after the introduction of GE crops, it is estimated that pesticide use in the United States increased by over 300 million pounds. Also, in 2008 GE crops required over 25 percent more pesticides per acre, compared to their non-GE counterparts.[33] In a replay of the 1960s and 70s, mainstream scientists are thus once again documenting adverse environmental and health effects from an overreliance on synthetic pesticides, and are making renewed calls to move agriculture towards more ecologically-based, low-input production systems.

Dr. Héctor Valenzuela is a Professor and Vegetable Crops Extension Specialist at the University of Hawai'i at Manoa, CTAHR, Department of Plant and Environmental Protection Sciences. He received his Ph.D. in Vegetable Crops from the University of Florida, and BS and MS in Agronomy and Horticulture/IPM at Washington State University. Dr. Valenzuela conducts statewide educational programs and field research on sustainable agriculture and small-scale organic farming.

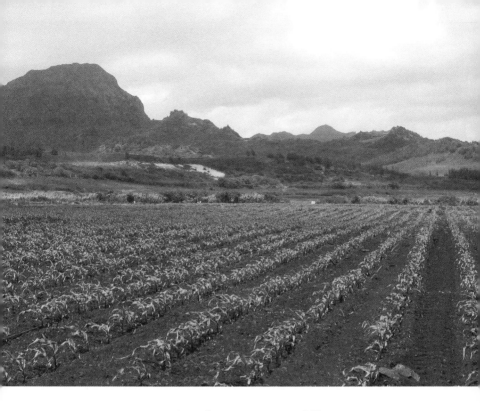

GMOs in Hawai'i
The Big Picture

Nancy Redfeather

There is a global gold rush happening, and the gold is life itself. The largest chemical companies in the world, makers of dangerous toxins which persist and migrate across borders, have added agricultural genetic engineering to their corporate business plans and are busy mining and manipulating the natural genetic resources and foods of the Earth. Just as land once owned in common was expropriated by the wealthy, so the "genetic commons" are now up for grabs. Due to changes in international patent laws, corporations can now patent, own and license microorganisms, plants and animals, and the genes they contain. Even humans are not exempt; at last count, 20 percent of human genes have now been patented in the United States alone.

These corporations are the new "genetic engineers." With full support and financial assistance of federal and state governments, land-grant universities (such as the University of Hawai'i at Manoa), and their regulators the EPA, FDA, and USDA, the rush is on to control the seeds of life.[1] Whoever controls the seed, controls the food and, ultimately, the people. Many of these corporations (Monsanto, Dow, Dupont/Pioneer, Syngenta, etc.) use Hawaiian soils to test their new genetically altered agricultural crops. Hawai'i has the distinction of being the world's center for experimental testing, with no environmental assessments before or following a test. Although proponents of the technology claim that these field trials are the "most regulated" crops in the history of agriculture, this simply is not so. The EPA and FDA have no field inspectors in Hawai'i.

A December 2005 audit by the Office of the Inspector General of the USDA's approval and regulatory processes for GMO crops severely criticized every aspect of these so-called regulations, finding them to be insufficient and inadequate to properly protect the environment.[2] In Hawai'i, where we have more experimental field trials than anywhere else in the U.S., this report needs to be taken very seriously.

Why Hawai'i? We are the most isolated island chain in the world, and have a year-round growing season. Beginning in earnest in the mid-1990s, corporations were courted to come and set up shop here. The Hawai'i Legislature enacted laws to financially assist and protect these companies. These laws (Act 221 and now Act 215, meant to encourage high technology businesses in Hawai'i) provide investment capital, give tax subsidies, tax credits for research activities, exclude royalties from gross income and give tax exemptions on stock options. Which companies receive these benefits, and the exact amount of these benefits, is confidential business information (CBI) not available to Hawai'i's citizens.[3,4,5]

Hawai'i's taxpayers are helping to subsidize the world's largest corporations in their takeover and cornering of the world market on seeds, food and drugs grown in plants. While these companies say that they wish only to feed the world, alleviate pain and suffering, and make agriculture more "environmentally friendly," the reality is very different.

For instance, over 80 percent of the world's GM crops are designed to withstand repeated sprayings with powerful herbicides – increasing chemical use – and are used mainly to feed animals, not people.

At this time, developing countries are being pressured by the U.S. government to pass new "intellectual property" laws that prevent farmers from saving and reusing, trading, or selling seeds. Worldwide there are countries, including the United States, that are seeking to make farmers into seed consumers dependent on external sources instead of reusing farm saved seed. Traditional rights for farmers as breeders, producers of seed, seed exchangers and seed buyers are disappearing and being replaced with "intellectual property" laws, which seek to protect and create new markets for GMO and other patented seed. In Iraq, Order 81, enacted by the U.S. government, prohibits the farmers of Iraq who have traditionally saved 97 percent of their agricultural seed, from saving "protected" seed, provided by multinational companies. These laws seek to remove 10,000-year-old "farmers rights," which allow farmers to save a portion of every crop they grow for seed, a basic foundation for self-reliance and of subsistence agriculture.

Hawai'i's genetic engineers are the University of Hawai'i (UH) at Manoa and the Pacific Basin Agricultural Research Center (PBARC), based in Hilo. These federally and state-funded institutions, whose mission is to assist the farmers of Hawai'i and the Pacific Rim, along with the Hawai'i Agricultural Research Center (HARC) on O'ahu, are busy altering and claiming ownership of our tropical fruits, vegetables, beverages, nuts and herbs. UH is now "expected" to develop intellectual property to generate revenues. Student programs in tropical agriculture are being replaced with agricultural genetic engineering courses, when most people in Hawai'i would agree that UH is perfectly situated to be the center of ecological/sustainable tropical research and programs for the farmers of the Pacific Basin.

Some of Hawai'i's leaders have bought into the myth that biotech agriculture is the wave of the future, seemingly oblivious to enormous opposition from consumers, food companies and export markets.

Many people are questioning the long-term wisdom of such a decision. Hawai'i stands at a crossroads. Either we continue to pursue the manipulation and ownership of the genes of life, or we turn our attention and our unique world perspective and knowledge of tropical agriculture to developing ecological/sustainable agricultural systems that will benefit Hawai'i's farmers and the peoples of the Hawaiian islands, who will always need to eat. Let's put our resources and public funds to work for everyone, developing agricultural systems that benefit the people and cherish and steward the 'āina.

Nancy Redfeather is a teacher and gardener. She is the Program Director for the Hawai'i Island School Garden Network, a project of The Kohala Center. She is also a member of the Statewide Hawai'i Farm to School and School Garden Hui and the Hawai'i School Garden Task Force. She is the Director of the Hawai'i Public Seed Initiative and on the Board of the Organic Seed and Trade Association (OSGATA). She lives with her husband Gerry on their organic farm at Kawanui, Hawai'i and enjoys growing and preparing locally produced foods.

Gaining Ground in the Courts
Legal Conflicts Around GE Crops

Paul H. Achitoff and George A. Kimbrell

U.S. federal oversight of genetically engineered (GE) crops[1] can be charitably described as limited, or more accurately, as a failure. Over the past fifteen years, commercial approval has opened the door to the planting of millions of transgenic acres, yet the environmental and health impacts of this widespread change in our agricultural landscape were not being studied or regulated. The vast majority of these crops are engineered to be resistant to herbicides, namely Monsanto's Roundup. The impacts from these crop systems include the transgenic contamination of natural plants and non-GE crops, the creation of herbicide-resistant "superweeds," and the dramatic increase in the overall herbicidal load on the environment. The U.S. Department of Agriculture (USDA), entrusted with chief responsibility for testing and regulating these transgenic plants, has proven unable to contain them, and as a result they have caused significant economic harm and transgenic pollution of both conventional and wild plant species. Independent government investigations and reports, courts, and even Congress have found USDA's practices woefully inadequate.

Over the last half-dozen years, oversight of GE crops has in large part been defined by public interest litigation, on behalf of farmers, consumers, and environmental groups. These cases include a 2010 U.S. Supreme Court case, the first one about GE crops to be decided by the United States' highest court. This body of precedent, discussed below, has permanently altered the former legal landscape, improving it in several fundamental ways, although there remains much work to be done.

Genetically Engineered Biopharmaceutical Crops: *Center for Food Safety v. Johanns,* 451 F. Supp. 2d 1165 (D. Haw. 2006) (*Hawai'i Biopharm*).

Hawai'i Biopharm was one of the first cases to hold that USDA has a legal duty to analyze the environmental and socioeconomic impacts of permitting the field testing of experimental GE crops, including the contamination of

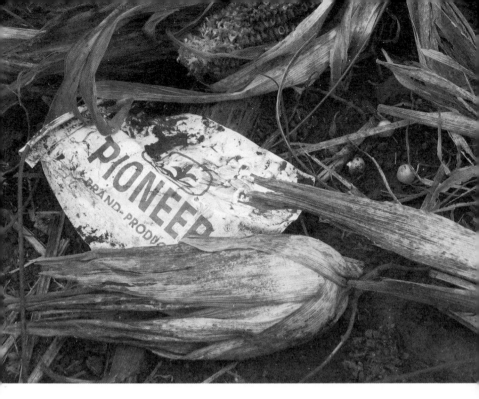

organic, conventional and wild plants. It was also one of the first cases to hold that the escape of transgenic DNA from engineered plants to natural plants and animals is a form of environmental harm.

USDA had issued permits to ProdiGene, Monsanto, Garst Seed and the Hawai'i Agriculture Research Center (HARC) authorizing each of them to plant genetically engineered corn or sugarcane using over 330 tons of seed in at least nine different locations on O'ahu, Maui, Kaua'i, Moloka'i, and Lana'i, on over 816 acres – more than 1.25 square miles of plantings. These experimental crops, using genes derived from some eighteen different donor organisms, including humans, were designed to produce two dozen different pharmaceutical proteins – drugs – including:

- human granulocyte macrophage stimulating factor
- human monoclonal antibodies
- experimental AIDS vaccine using glycoprotein 120
- experimental hepatitis B vaccine
- aprotinin
- trypsin
- proinsulin

- experimental transmissible gastroenteritis virus ("TGEV") (swine diarrhea) vaccine

The companies growing these experimental crops (known as a group as GE "biopharm" crops) hoped to reduce their cost of producing these drugs by using open fields instead of laboratories, and engineering the plants to grow the drugs instead of having to synthesize them. They also hoped to eliminate the cost of the security measures typically used to isolate such production from the public or competitors – such as fences, locks, security guards, or surveillance systems – by relying on public ignorance, and refusing to inform the public of the nature of the crops or their locations.

No tolerances (maximum safe exposure levels) existed for any of these proteins; no human exposure was legally allowable. Yet all of these experiments used plants that are widely eaten by humans and animals, are virtually indistinguishable from the corn and sugarcane that is safe to eat, and capable of cross-pollinating edible crops. According to scientific experts, exposure to even minute quantities of many of these proteins could cause serious health problems in humans and animals. For example, Dr. David Schubert, professor at the Salk Institute of Biological Studies and head of the Institute's Cellular Neurobiology Laboratory, pointed out that if workers harvesting or processing the AIDS vaccine-producing corn inhaled the corn pollen or dust, their immune systems might become unresponsive to AIDS infections, "with potentially lethal consequences." Dr. Schubert noted that exposure to prothrombin (a blood-clotting protein) or monoclonal antibodies may cause autoimmune disorders, and exposure to proinsulin may cause Type 1 diabetes. Aprotinin is a blood-clotting protein derived from cows, and is known to cause anaphylactic shock in humans and pancreatic cancer in animals. It also is toxic to honey bees that consume pollen containing aprotinin.

Not surprisingly, a broad spectrum of interests, including Consumers' Union, the Union of Concerned Scientists, and the National Academy of Sciences expressed concerns about the risk of such tests contaminating the food supply and environment, and the National Food Processors Association and Grocery Manufacturers of America, expressed concerns about food contamination and liability.

The permits allowed these companies to plant these experimental crops in open-air fields, with no requirement that the fields be marked or people be informed of what was being grown or where it was being grown. In fact,

USDA adamantly refused to disclose where any of the fields were located other than the islands where planting had been authorized, because the companies claimed the locations were "confidential business information," or "CBI." Extensive litigation resulting in court orders was required to force the government to disclose the locations, and even then only the plaintiffs' attorneys were given access, subject to strict requirements that they never disclose the information to anyone else. It can be said, however, that one site was near a school. Monsanto's many test sites were scattered along West Maui's Honoapi'ilani Highway. Some plots were near areas that are home to dozens of endangered and endemic species. Wind carries corn pollen long distances, and the corn plots themselves were accessible to wildlife. No warning signs alerted passersby to the nature of the crops, which looked like any other corn.

The National Environmental Policy Act (NEPA) requires agencies to broadly analyze the environmental effects of their actions, including issuance of permits, in an Environmental Assessment (EA) or Environmental Impact Statement (EIS), and the Endangered Species Act (ESA) requires assessment of impacts on threatened and endangered species and designated critical habitat. Yet USDA failed to perform any analysis whatsoever of the possible effects of outdoor growing of these experimental crops on any aspect of human health, the environment, or protected species. Accordingly, in late 2003, Center For Food Safety, KAHEA; Friends of the Earth, and Pesticide Action Network – North America, represented by attorneys from Earthjustice and Center for Food Safety, sued to challenge USDA's failure to comply with these laws. The Biotechnology Industry Organization (BIO), a trade association of biotech companies, intervened on the government's side. In August 2006, the federal district court in Hawai'i ruled that the government had, in fact, violated NEPA and acted in "utter disregard" of the ESA by failing to perform the required analyses before issuing the permits.

Genetically Engineered Grasses: *International Center for Technology Assessment v. Johanns,* 473 F. Supp. 2d 9 (D.D.C. 2007) *motion to dismiss appeal granted*, No. 07-5238, (D.C. Cir. Mar. 17, 2008) (*GE Grasses*).

In the *GE Grasses* case, environmentalists and public interest organizations[2] challenged USDA's approval of numerous experimental open-air field trials of genetically engineered, herbicide resistant grasses created by Monsanto and licensed to Scotts.[3] The case was one of the first to focus specifically on "standing" (or the right to go to court and seek relief) for environmental organizations challenging field testing of GE crops, holding that the risk of contamination and other environmental harms was sufficient to challenge the USDA's decision.

The GE grasses were engineered with resistance to Monsanto's herbicide, Roundup, and intended for eventual commercial use on lawns and golf courses. As in *Hawai'i Biopharm*, USDA had again failed to undertake any NEPA assessment whatsoever of the field testings' potential impacts. The plaintiffs argued that the GE grass would escape the test plots and threatened biodiversity, through transgenic contamination of natural grasses, as well as further threaten the surrounding natural habitats of other plants. USDA, and Scotts, which intervened to defend USDA's decision, argued that there was no meaningful risk of escape and even if there was, USDA was not required to analyze its impacts.

A federal district court for the District of Columbia disagreed, concluding that the USDA could not approve field trials of the GE grasses without environmental review under NEPA. As a consequence, field trials of the GE grasses halted in 2007. However, during the course of the litigation it was discovered that the transgenic grass, which is pollinated by wind, had already escaped one of the test sites in eastern Oregon and contaminated a protected national grassland over a dozen miles away.

USDA blamed Scotts for the wild grassland contamination, required the company to exterminate the escapees, and fined them a half-million dollars. Unfortunately this was not the end of the story: in fall of 2010, even though no further field testing had been allowed, eastern Oregon farmers found new (until then undiscovered) populations of the GE grasses, thriving in the wild. USDA did not publicly disclose this, but it was revealed during cross-examination of a USDA official in another GE crop case in late 2010. Scotts continues to work with USDA and the Oregon Department of Agriculture to try locate and exterminate these feral GE grasses.

Although USDA had previously considered Scotts' petition for commercial approval of the grasses, after the *GE Grasses* field trial case the agency has never subsequently proposed that they be approved for commercialization. In 2010, the U.S. Fish and Wildlife Service (FWS) concluded that allowing the commercialization of Roundup Ready bentgrass could cause the extinction of two endangered plants in Oregon because the GE grass would spread the transgenic resistance to wild relatives, which would then take over the species' critical habitat and be impossible to eradicate.

Genetically Engineered Alfalfa: *Geertson Seed Farms v. Johanns*, 2007 WL 518624 (N.D. Cal. Feb. 13, 2007), *affirmed*, 541 F.3d 938 (9th Cir. 2008) (*GE Alfalfa*).

In *GE Alfalfa*, environmentalists and organic and conventional farmers,[4] represented by attorneys from Center for Food Safety, challenged USDA's unconditional approval of Monsanto's GE "Roundup Ready" alfalfa after conducting only a cursory environmental review. Alfalfa is the fourth most widely grown crop in the United States (at approximately 20 million acres), behind corn, soybeans, and wheat; it is grown in every state. GE alfalfa is another crop engineered to withstand direct application of glyphosate, the active ingredient in herbicide formulations manufactured and sold by the commercial name Roundup by Monsanto. Because growers can apply the chemical without being concerned that it may harm their crops, the use of Roundup Ready crops has dramatically increased use of glyphosate, which is now found in soil, groundwater, surface waters and even rain. Glyphosate, like all herbicides, is toxic to plants, animals and humans.

Overreliance on applications of glyphosate has caused glyphosate resistant weeds to evolve. Although the herbicide kills almost all weeds, a few individual weed plants will be naturally resistant. These will survive, reproduce, and take over the field. As a result of this selection pressure created by constant Roundup use, about a dozen species of glyphosate resistant weeds now infest millions of acres of United States farmland as well as land in other countries growing Roundup Ready crops, causing farmers to apply older, even more toxic herbicides, or even resort to hoeing by hand.

GE alfalfa is the first genetically engineered perennial and bee-pollinated crop. Bees can cross pollinate at distances of many miles, posing significant seed contamination impacts. Alfalfa can also thrive as a feral plant, ubiquitous in roadsides, irrigation ditches, and range lands across the western United States, acting as a transgenic "bridge" that further contaminates the wild.

Organic businesses were extremely concerned because alfalfa is considered the "Queen of Forages," and is the main feed ingredient of the organic dairy industry. Federal organic standards prohibit the use of genetic engineering, and all organic animal husbandry requires 100 percent organic feed. United States organic consumers expect that organic products will be GE-free, as its exclusion is one of the main reasons people buy organic. The United States also has a thriving 200 million dollar-a-year alfalfa hay and seed export market, mostly to GE-sensitive countries.

Finally, current conventional alfalfa production uses little or no pesticides, so adoption of the herbicide-resistant variety would lead to massive increases in pesticide use. Replacing conventional with Roundup Ready alfalfa on millions of acres would dramatically increase the crop's cumulative herbicide load on the environment, in a crop that is considered important wildlife habitat. Alfalfa also is commonly rotated with other Roundup Ready crops, raising concerns that adding yet another herbicide-dependent cropping system could worsen the glyphosate-resistant weed epidemic.

The *GE Alfalfa* case marked the first time that a federal district court held illegal USDA's commercialization approval for a GE crop without preparing a full Environmental Impact Statement (EIS) under NEPA. Remarkably, in over fifteen years of approving GE crops, USDA had never before undertaken an EIS for any GE crop approval. The GE Alfalfa court concluded that transgenic contamination of organic and conventional alfalfa seed and plants was a significant environmental impact triggering the EIS requirement. It also concluded that USDA failed to consider the impact on farmers of contamination of non-genetically engineered alfalfa, and whether Roundup Ready alfalfa will increase the development of glyphosate resistant weeds and increase overall pesticide use. These were all precedent-setting findings. The court then vacated, or set aside, USDA's decision to commercialize Monsanto's Roundup Ready alfalfa and issued a permanent injunction that halted the planting and sale of the crop nationwide pending USDA's issuance and preparation of a full EIS.

The *GE Alfalfa* decision was the first to hold that economic impacts on farmers resulting from contamination, or even just the risk of contamination, were cognizable injuries that required analysis, and for which equitable relief could be granted. These impacts include lost markets, lost organic certification, and lost reputation. But more fundamentally, the decision created important precedent in holding that contamination of seeds caused the loss of the farmers' and consumers' right to choose the crop of their choice, and was an irreparable injury.

GE Crops at the Supreme Court: *Monsanto Company v. Geertson Seed Farms,* 130 S.Ct. 2743 (2010).

Monsanto, holder of the intellectual property rights to Roundup Ready alfalfa, and its licensee, Forage Genetics, both of which had intervened in the case, appealed the district court's issuance of the injunction that imposed a nationwide ban on the sale and planting of the crop. The Supreme Court set aside the injunction, but did so innocuously, holding that it was simply unnecessary in light of the other remedy granted, the vacatur, which independently halted the alfalfa's planting (by reverting it to its previous status as a "regulated article"). The Court also held that USDA had the authority to restrict GE crops to prevent contamination and other agronomic harms.

Finally, the Court also declined to reach or agree with a number of other far-reaching arguments that Monsanto had vigorously advocated, many of which would have significantly weakened or eliminated the judicial review of GE crop regulation (and environmental law generally).

The case marked the first Supreme Court case to deal with the impacts of genetically engineered crops. It affirmed in the legal landscape the earlier lower court determinations discussed above that: 1) transgenic contamination of conventional and organic seed (as well the risk of it and onerous measures needed to protect against it) is a both an environmental as well as economic injury; 2) the risk of contamination is a type of injury that can give a plaintiff standing to sue; and 3) GE crop approvals may be set aside for failure to perform a proper review of their impacts, including transgenic contamination, and may be limited by the agency to prevent these impacts.

After the Supreme Court's decision, in early 2011, USDA finished its court-ordered EIS on GE alfalfa, which ran several thousand pages. The agency's unprecedented analysis of the GE crop's impacts showed that commercializing GE alfalfa would likely cause significant environmental, agronomic and economic damage through contamination, herbicide resistant weeds and massively increased use of herbicides. Organic farmers and businesses, exporters of conventional alfalfa and alfalfa seed, and native ecosystems, including dozens of endangered species, would be harmed.

Nonetheless, USDA, after considering and recommending a restricted approval with mandatory conditions to mitigate contamination, decided to unconditionally approve GE alfalfa again, allowing it to be grown anywhere without any oversight or restrictions. In March 2011, the GE alfalfa plaintiff farmers and environmental organizations filed suit again, challenging that decision. A federal court affirmed the USDA's decision in January 2012. That decision is currently on appeal in the Ninth Circuit Court of Appeals.

Genetically Engineered Sugar Beets: *Ctr. for Food Safety v. Vilsack*, 2009 WL 3047227 (N.D. Cal. 2009); 734 F.Supp.2d 948 (N.D. Cal. 2010); *appeal voluntarily dismissed*, No. 10-17335 (9th Cir. 2011) (*GE Beets I*).

Sugar beets account for about half of the sugar produced in the United States. In 2005, APHIS granted a petition submitted by Monsanto and a German company, KWS SAAT AG, to allow growers to plant Roundup Ready sugar beets (RRSB), genetically engineered to tolerate dousing with glyphosate herbicide.

Much RRSB seed[5] is produced in Oregon's fertile Willamette Valley, where seed for related organic crops also is grown. Beet seed is carried for miles by the wind, and organic seed producers understandably worry about cross-pollination, which could destroy their businesses and is expensive to try to prevent, costly to detect, and virtually impossible to remove once it happens.

In early 2008, Center for Food Safety, Sierra Club, Organic Seed Alliance and High Mowing Organic Seeds sued USDA in the federal district court in San Francisco, challenging the agency's decision to allow RRSB to be grown anywhere, without any restrictions or oversight. The plaintiffs also alleged USDA had violated NEPA by failing to prepare an EIS, instead preparing a cursory EA which concluded that growing RRSB and spraying it with glyphosate would have "no significant impact" on human health or the environment. Monsanto, Syngenta, the companies producing RRSB seed, and companies growing and processing sugar beets all intervened to defend the government's position that no meaningful analysis was required and that, even if it was, the industry should be allowed to continue growing the crop throughout the northern United States while APHIS belatedly performed its legal duties.

After three years of litigation, the court in August 2010 found that contamination by engineered crops threatens the livelihoods of organic and conventional farmers, and deprives consumers of the ability to choose the foods they prefer. The court agreed with the plaintiffs that USDA had unlawfully allowed RRSB on the market, and that before doing so again it had to prepare an EIS examining, among other things, contamination risks and the effects of glyphosate use with the crop.

Center For Food Safety v. Vilsack, et al., 753 F. Supp. 2d 1051(N.D. Cal. 2010), *vacated and remanded*, 636 F.3d 1166 (9th Cir. 2011) (*GE Beets II*); *Ctr. for Food Safety v. Vilsack*, No. C 11-00586 JSB (D.D.C. filed Feb. 23, 2011) (*GE Beets III*).

The government and the sugar beet industry were not willing to halt production of RRSB regardless of the court's order, and created a scheme to allow production to continue without pause, despite the lack of any meaningful environmental review. Only three weeks after the court declared unlawful the RRSB deregulation and failure to prepare an EIS, USDA issued field trial permits allowing the industry to plant hundreds of more acres of RRSB to produce seed.

APHIS failed to assess any environmental impacts of either the seed crop or the root crop that the seed crop was intended to enable the industry to plant later. For example, when the seed crop flowers and the male plants shed billions of grains of wind-carried pollen to fertilize the female plants in order to create seed, organic and conventional farmers in the Willamette Valley face possible cross-pollination of their own crops; sugar beets, Swiss chard, and table beets are all the same species and can all pollinate each other. The government claimed no prior evaluation of this (or any) risk was necessary, because it intended to prepare an Environmental Assessment while the seed crop was growing, and issue it before the plants flowered. Of course, the law requires such assessments before the government allows an activity to occur, not after; obviously, USDA judgment in its belated EA would likely be affected by the investment in the seed crop it had already allowed industry to make months before.

The same groups therefore went back to court and in September 2010, filed *GE Beets II*, a new lawsuit challenging USDA's permits for the RRSB seed crop. They asked the court to issue an injunction to stop the planting, but the crop was planted within a few days. The court subsequently concluded the crop had been planted unlawfully and ordered it destroyed. On appeal, however, this order was reversed and the seed crop was allowed to mature.

APHIS then "partially deregulated" the RRSB seed and root crop subject to some restrictions it claimed would prevent contamination, and issued a belated EA. The government argued the challenge to the permits was now moot, and the court agreed, dismissing the plaintiffs' case. That dismissal is on appeal in the Ninth Circuit Court of Appeals as of this writing.

The plaintiff groups then filed another lawsuit to challenge the partial deregulation, and that suit is now pending in a Washington, D.C. federal court. In June 2012, APHIS issued the EIS the *Beets I* court had ordered it to prepare, and deregulated RRSB permanently. As of this writing the court has yet to decide whether the deregulation and EIS made the plaintiffs' claims moot.

Conclusion

Prior to the ground-breaking genetically engineered crop litigation discussed above, in the United States, there was no meaningful environmental review of the significant adverse environmental and economic impacts of GE crops before their approval or testing. Seed diversity and integrity was at unabated risk, because transgenic contamination of seeds was not considered an injury. Cross-pollination or seed mixing, causing transfer of foreign DNA to organic, conventional, or natural wild plants was known by the Orwellian term "adventitious presence." Because there supposedly was no injury, neither farmers nor environmental advocates had "standing" to even seek redress in court, let alone be granted relief. USDA had no obligation to even consider limiting the planting of GE crops when approving them. Similarly, weed resistance and increased herbicide impacts proliferated without consideration or analysis.

Over the last half dozen years, the above body of precedent altered the legal landscape in several fundamental ways. For example, transgenic contamination of seeds and plants is now established as harm for which farmers and environmental advocates can seek redress in our courts, can prevail on the merits of their claim, and can be granted injunctive and declaratory relief. More fundamentally, the courts have recognized seed contamination irreparably injures farmers' right to choose to sow the crop of their choice, and consumers' right to choose the foods they eat. USDA can no longer ignore these risks, and must now analyze them. Governmental agencies also must now consider, for the first time, restrictions on the commercial approval of such crops.

Paul Achitoff and George Kimbrell are attorneys with Earthjustice and the Center for Food Safety, respectively, which have co-counseled on most of the litigation described in this chapter.

Agency Definitions and Jurisdictions

USDA regulates transgenic crops under the Plant Protection Act (PPA), 6 U.S.C. §§ 7701-7772, which provides the agency with broad authority to "prohibit or restrict ... movement in interstate commerce of any plant" as necessary to prevent either "plant pest" or "noxious weed" harms.[6] The statute's multifaceted purpose is to protect not only agriculture, but the "environment, and economy of the United States" through the "detection, control, eradication, suppression, prevention, or retardation" of these harms.[7] The PPA defines these harms expansively. A "noxious weed" harm is "any plant or plant product that can directly or indirectly injure or cause damage to crops ... or other interests of agriculture, ... the natural resources of the United States, the public health, or the environment."[8] "Plant pest" means: "any living stage [of a list of organisms] that can directly or indirectly injure, cause damage to, or cause disease in any plant or plant product."[9] GE plants are classified as "regulated articles" that cannot be grown commercially. The agency prescribes how, if at all, they may be "introduce[d]" into the environment.[10] Developers seeking to commercialize a transgenic plant must petition The Animal and Plant Health Inspection Service (APHIS) for "deregulation," which the agency can grant "in whole or in part."[11]

Herbicide tolerant crops account for the large majority of all GE crop acreage worldwide.[12] In most cases, these crops have been engineered to survive being doused with the herbicide glyphosate, which Monsanto Company produces and sells as Roundup. Monsanto also engineers most of the herbicide tolerant crops themselves and patents the seeds. It then markets the seed and Roundup together as the two components of a "Roundup Ready crop system." A farmer using this system pays a substantial premium for the patented seed so that he may spray Roundup on his fields even while the crop is growing; glyphosate is a broad-spectrum, non-selective herbicide toxic to virtually all plants, just not the engineered crop.[13]

In the absence of any limitations on these crop systems and their concomitant harms, non-profit groups have challenged some GE crop deregulations by pointing out that USDA has allowed the crops on the market without complying with the PPA. For example, herbicide tolerant GE crops plainly meet the legal definitions of harms covered by the PPA, giving USDA ample power, and obligation, to regulate them in order to protect agriculture and the environment. Recent litigation has also centered on two other federal statutes. Whenever a federal agency takes action – which may include issuing a permit or granting a petition to deregulate a GE crop – the agency must comply with at least two environmental laws: the National Environmental

Policy Act (NEPA), 42 U.S.C. § 4321, et seq., and the Endangered Species Act (ESA), 16 U.S.C. § 1531, et seq.

NEPA "protect[s] the environment by requiring that federal agencies carefully weigh environmental considerations and consider potential alternatives to the proposed action before the government launches any major federal action."[14] It requires that before an agency acts, it must determine whether its action may have a significant effect on the environment. If the agency is not sure, it may prepare an Environmental Assessment (EA). This document examines the effects of the action as well as alternatives to it, and is circulated for comment by the public and other agencies. The analysis must include effects on the environment, such as water or air quality, on plants and animals, and on socioeconomic impacts that are interrelated with these and other kinds of environmental effects.

If the agency reasonably concludes that its action will have no significant environmental effects, it prepares a Finding of No Significant Impact (FONSI), and may proceed with its action. If it concludes that its action may have a significant impact, it must prepare an Environmental Impact Statement (EIS). An EIS presents a more lengthy and detailed analysis of impacts and alternatives than an EA. Once an agency prepares an EIS that complies with all legal requirements, such as scientific reliability, breadth of scope and consideration of reasonable alternatives, the agency may select among the alternatives and proceed.

The ESA generally prohibits anyone from harming species listed as endangered or threatened, or the habitats that have been designated as critical to the species' survival or recovery. Section 7(a)(2) of the ESA, 16 U.S.C. § 1536(a)(2), requires that before a federal agency acts, it must examine whether its action may affect any threatened or endangered species, or any critical habitat.[15] If the agency determines that its action may have any such effect, it must consult with the agencies Congress created to exercise expertise concerning wildlife conservation: the U.S. Fish and Wildlife Service (in the case of terrestrial species) and/or the National Marine Fisheries Service (NMFS) (in the case of marine species). Unless these agencies confirm in writing that the agency action will not adversely affect any protected species or habitat, the agency must formally consult with these expert agencies. This process results in the expert agency drafting a Biological Opinion that determines whether the agency action is likely to jeopardize the continued existence of any threatened or endangered species, or adversely modify any critical habitat. If the assessment concludes that this is likely and the agency proceeds anyway, it risks violating the ESA's strict prohibition on harming protected species.

| FIELD WAS SPRAYED ON: | DATE **5/26** | TIME **10:40** |
| DO NOT ENTER BEFORE: | DATE **5/27** | TIME **10:40** |

PESTICIDE(S) APPLIED:
PLEASE CIRCLE

RE: ~~24HRS~~ 48HRS

PROWL	ACCENT	~~ATRAZIN~~
BANVEL	CABARYL	~~LASSO~~
BUCTRIL	TILT	LIBERTY
DIMETHOATE	~~LORSBAN~~	QUADRIS
ASANA	ROUND-UP	
OTHER:		

DANGER
PESTICIDES

Public Health and the Regulation of GMOs

Lorrin Pang, MD, MPH

Each day, many new foods, drugs, vaccines and diagnostics are developed that could affect our health. Hidden among the potential miracles are potential disasters. Ideally, society should be able to distinguish between the two and minimize the risk to health and environment.

But these are complicated products, full of uncertainty, and the average person does not have the time, training or interest to research, or even follow the evaluation of each new product. Thus, we delegate this responsibility to the regulators – agencies that should follow time-tested principles and methods to evaluate the risks and benefits of new products.

In general the Food and Drug Administration (FDA) is responsible for health, the Environmental Protection Agency (EPA) for environmental risks and the U.S. Department of Agriculture (USDA) for risk to agriculture.

Poorly conducted regulation is worse than no regulation at all because it will lead to a false sense of security. One of our key regulatory agencies, the FDA, has come under repeated criticism for allowing those with ties to industry to bias their decisions.

GMOs are a very complex and novel product. According to the U.S. National Academy of Sciences, they have a greater potential for unintended health effects compared to non-GMO foods.[1] Those defending the industry will often misrepresent this citation, stating that the side effects are "similar." Qualitatively this may be true, but quantitatively GMOs are riskier. They require a higher level of safety testing than non-GMO foods. But how much extra testing should be required? And who will decide? For reasons cited above, the testing criteria should *not* be defined by those with conflicts of interest in the issue.

What is regulation and who does it?

The essence of regulation for food and drugs really lies with a group of about a dozen scientists and lay people who review the results from a prescribed sequence of studies. These studies include proof of a method of manufacturing that produces consistent product, laboratory testing, animal trials, human trials and, finally, post-marketing surveys.

In the course of the studies, one hopes to obtain results that are scientifically valid as well as to minimize risks to animals and human subjects. Yet with the exception of a handful of human studies, the GMO industry relies only on minimal animal studies to screen products for safety. In the case of other drugs and vaccines we have seen many products that cleared animal studies, only to have toxicity detected in humans.

The drug industry often cites post-marketing safety data. However, it is nearly impossible to evaluate post-marketing safety if products such as GMOs are not labeled. Even when products are identified (for example, asbestos, lead or tobacco) it may take decades to detect their harmful effects. According to the World Health Organization (WHO) assistant director-general Kerstin Leitner, "At this point, we have no evidence to say that it is dangerous to consume food products that contain GMOs, but at the same time we also don't know its negative side. So, we have to say that we do not know the adverse health effects of GM food," (Bangkok Post, October 13, 2004). Industry supporters have often attributed statements to the WHO that potential benefits of GMO methods far outweigh the risks. For drugs and vaccines this may be true – but only under the conditions of adequate regulatory safeguards.

In Hawai'i, the field testing of experimental crops puts workers and neighboring communities at risk. Crop type and location of field tests are not disclosed to the public, even those used for pharmaceutical (as opposed to food) production. We have received assurances from the industry and their supporters that proper safeguards are in place – but, as mentioned above, those who define these safety standards should not have conflicts of interest.

Because of the novelty of the genetic mutations created; our present ignorance of genome structure and function; and the complex relationship of genetic manipulations to human health and environmental effects – there may be a multitude of future consequences and interactions that we have not even begun to imagine. Side effects may include toxins, cancers, allergies, antibiotic resistance and anaphylaxis reactions. It is unknown if genetically engineered mutations can directly or indirectly (via viruses or bacteria) incorporate into the genes of humans. Especially disconcerting are chronic exposures to either high doses (foods) or low doses (aerosolized) of GMO products, which are life forms with the potential for uncontrolled contamination and difficulty of recall.

Yet it is clear that by conscientiously applying regulatory guidelines to the process of product assessment – guidelines that are widely accepted in other fields but are being overlooked in the rush to bring new GMO products to market – potential side effects can be mitigated.

These regulatory guidelines and policies should include:

- **Precautionary Principle.** All products are assumed to be ineffective and toxic until proven otherwise. Theoretical arguments only guide us as to what types of effects we should focus our monitoring on – otherwise general evaluations are conducted.
- **Conflicts of interest** by all who participate in safety reviews must be clearly documented and members are expected to limit their participation in areas where a conflict might arise. Often those with greatest conflicts will be the most indignant about having this pointed out.
- **Product evaluation** is done on a case-by-case basis. Even combinations of products (relevant to the promoter-gene-marker construct of GMOs) should be considered a "new" product warranting a new evaluation. Though one can hypothesize between products based on molecular

similarities, empirical tests are still required. Many "similar" products with vastly different side effects could not be predicted theoretically in hindsight – let alone in foresight. Conversely, if a regulatory agency has been shown to have a biased decision-making process for one product, the precautionary principle would indicate that all products might have been judged with bias.

- **Consistency of product must be shown** (within predetermined limits of contaminations) before studies can even begin. Some GMO products (biolistic production) are potentially highly variable, which would make it difficult to conduct valid safety studies over time, with reproducible results.

- **Raw data of results must be reviewed.** A board that only looks at summaries done by other agencies really defeats the purpose of the board itself.

- **Approval is required from two boards:** one at the central level by those who make/sponsor the product and one at the local level, where the product is to be "tested." Locally, this approval may come in the form of an environmental impact statement or from a community based ethical review board if there is a health component to be assessed. No local reviews of this type have been conducted for GMO crops in Hawai'i. Boards should also determine who will be responsible for unintended effects and liability.

- **Control of enticement.** Benefits not directly related to the product itself (business opportunities, awarded grants) should not be considered "benefits" of the product.

Dr. Lorrin Pang, MD, MPH, graduated with honors from Princeton University in Chemistry and went on to get an MD and Masters in Public Health from Tulane University. Dr. Pang worked with the Walter Reed Institute of Research and the World Health Organization for 20 years doing research in Tropical Diseases before returning to Maui in 2000. Since then, he has served as the District Health Officer for Maui County and is a consultant for the World Health Organization and one of the world's largest pharmaceutical firms, Glaxo-Smith-Kline. He has published more than 50 research articles in medical and public health journals regarding drugs, vaccines and diagnostic tests. Dr. Pang writes here as a private citizen.

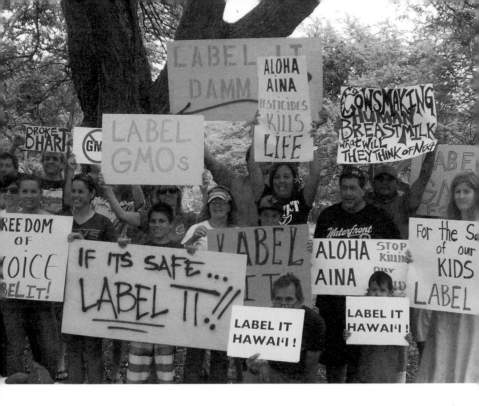

GMO Labeling Legislation
Breaking Open the Policy Door

Mary Lacques

In 2012, nearly one million registered California voters signed petition papers to place a Citizen's Initiative on the November ballot that would require mandatory labeling of genetically engineered (GE) foods. Proposition 37, "The Right to Know Initiative," although defeated by a 45 million dollar lobbying push by the GE industry, was one more flash point in policy debate that has been simmering for years in state legislatures and county governments around the country.

It appears that a majority of American consumers would embrace a national GE labeling law; a national poll by the Mellman Group conducted in February 2012 found that 91 percent of those questioned favored labeling of GE foods. What's more, these results were consistent within two percentage points among Independents, Republicans and Democrats.[1]

Results from a 2007 University of Hawai'i survey showed that 72 percent of Hawai'i residents said that labeling of GE foods was "very" important, while another 13 percent said it was "somewhat" important.[2] Hawai'i has a history of elected officials at the national level supporting legislation for the labeling of GE food. In 1999, Congresswoman Patsy Mink signed on to the Bonior/Kucinich U.S. House labeling letter to the Food and Drug Administration (FDA), which called for the labeling of GE foods.[3] Congresswoman Mink was a co-sponsor of H.R. 3377, The Genetically Engineered Food Right to Know Act, which required "that food that contains genetically engineered material ... be labeled accordingly." Mink also cosponsored H.R. 713 to require the Secretary of Agriculture to complete a report regarding the safety and monitoring of GE foods. In March of 2012, Senator Daniel Akaka, along with 54 other members of Congress, signed on to a bicameral letter addressed to the FDA asking the agency to require the labeling of GE foods.[4] In June of 2012, Senators Akaka and Inouye voted in favor of an amendment reaffirming the rights of states to pursue their own labeling of GE food laws.[5]

In Hawai'i, numerous GE labeling bills have been introduced in recent years. In 2011 Maui, Kaua'i and Hawai'i Counties all passed labeling resolutions, followed by Honolulu County in May of 2012. In 2012 alone, *twelve* GE labeling bills were introduced at the Hawai'i State Legislature, but both the House and Senate Agriculture Committee Chairs refused to schedule a hearing for any of them.[6] It is up to us Hawai'i residents, as consumers and registered voters, to assert our influence and insist that we are guaranteed the right to choose whether we would like to feed GE foods to our families or not.

If local producers are able to affix a sticker to Hawai'i-grown GE Rainbow Papaya prior to being shipped to Japan, we can certainly do the same for local consumers. We often hear that as consumers we have the ability to influence policy through "the power of the pocketbook," but we must have access to the information necessary to make these purchasing decisions. It is our responsibility as engaged citizens, and that of our elected officials, to demand this information. Labeling legislation does not argue whether the GE industry is good or bad, it simply argues for the right to choose – a core value of a healthy democratic society.

Mary Lacques is a teacher who works with economically challenged families on O'ahu. She is on the Board of Directors of Hawai'i SEED and is a founding member of Label it Hawai'i. She comes from a lineage of farmers and ranchers.

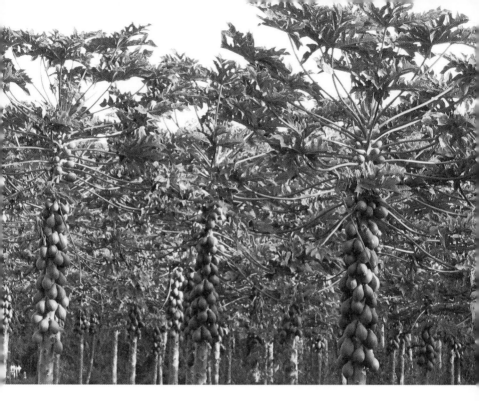

Papaya and Coffee
GMO "Solutions" Spell Market Disaster

Melanie Bondera

Hawai'i's major specialty crops were under attack by the biotech industry and our public research institutions. Our islands' significant farm products were being genetically transformed to create "agricultural solutions" which would have caused farmers no end of problems in production, marketing, liability, and loss of choice when real, sustainable solutions are usually attainable more quickly and cheaply.

Papaya

In 1998 the new GMO Papaya was released in Puna. It was heralded as the first GMO fruit and it would save an industry from a Ringspot virus epidemic. Rainbow and SunUp are the two varieties of GMO papayas that were released at that time, and, although these were indeed resistant to

Ringspot virus, both were plagued by Blackspot fungus and were immediately shut out of their most lucrative market: Japan.[1] Since then, we have lost half of the state's papaya farmers and the industry has continued to shrink.[2] Because the price point of the GMO papaya was always lower than the traditional varieties, and GMOs were never acceptable to consumers of whole foods, many GMO papaya farmers could not make a living, went out of business, or moved on to grow other crops.[3]

By 2004 evidence of rampant GMO papaya contamination was coming to light, so Hawai'i SEED did a study to analyze the extent of the contamination problem. Genetic ID of Fairfield, Iowa did composite PCR (polymerase chain reaction) tests for most islands and several case studies. Results showed that a shocking 50 percent of the non-GMO papaya seeds tested on the Big Island were contaminated with GMOs (see map, page 51). Even the University of Hawai'i (UH) seed source for non-GMO papaya in Waimanalo showed 1 percent contamination.[4] Conventional farmers had to test their trees and all of their shipments in order to keep their non-GMO papayas in Japan.[5] Organic farmers lost markets, seed lines, certifications and chopped down their trees in order to keep their organic integrity.[6] Clearly, the GMO Papaya has brought more problems for farmers than it has solved.

When consumers buy GMO Rainbow and SunUp papayas in the market, they are not labeled as GMO. When they take them home and cut them up for breakfast, the seeds are thrown in the compost – in essence, they plant them. Each GMO papaya you eat could "plant" up to 500 new GMO papaya trees. The primary cause of widespread contamination in Hawai'i is people, not pollen. UH requires growers to sign a contract, watch an informational video, and pay royalties when they lease GMO papaya seeds. But the university chooses to turn a blind eye to consumers unwittingly planting these trees. In 2011, after 13 years of lobbying Japan with a total of 13 million dollars of Hawai'i state taxpayer money, Japan's Ministry of Agriculture agreed to let GMO papayas in, but they must be labeled GMO. As these are some of the most anti-GMO consumers in the world, the product is not expected to sell well.

Dr. Dennis Gonsalves, head of the USDA Agricultural Research Service in Hilo, attempted to introduce GMO papayas in 13 other countries. Many of these countries actually field trialed the varieties, but none were commercialized. In Thailand, GMO crops were illegal and the government attempted to clean up the GMO contamination caused by a field trial in farmers' orchards. In the Philippines, the introduced GMO papayas got infected or died from a different strain of the Ringspot virus. In Jamaica, the GMO papaya project was cancelled because the UK is their main export market and consumers there have rejected GMO products. In Tanzania, the funding ran out before the field trial stage. Around the world, the simple method of roguing out virus-infected trees is still used effectively. The method of roguing infected plants was also used effectively in Puna, along with an intercropping method, for the production of non-GMO papayas for export to Japan.

Coffee

In 2002, Christine Sheppard, president of the Kona Coffee Council, became aware of the research on GMO coffees by UH and the Hawai'i Agriculture Research Center (HARC) that was nearing the field trial stage: attempts were being made to develop through genetic engineering a decaffeinated coffee, a nematode resistant coffee rootstock and a delayed ripening coffee that could be harvested green and sprayed with ethylene gas to complete the ripening. The Kona Coffee Council, along with four other farmers' groups, created a resolution protesting the release of these GMO coffees in the Kona region, based on the loss of markets they would likely experience. Hawai'i coffee is widely sold in the specialty and organic markets as well as in Japan and Europe. None of these markets tolerate GMOs.

"Kona coffee is recognized as one of the world's two best coffees," says Sheppard. "The coffee industry is rapidly changing and growing from a commodity product to a gourmet product. In an era of 'Specialty Coffees' we need to be unique. Fortunately, the Kona coffee pioneers blessed us with a historically significant variety that also produces great coffee. Introduction of GMO coffee plants would corrupt our heirloom stock, and it would no longer be the gourmet product that people have come to expect. Not only could this debase the flavor and quality of our coffee, but it would also make it unmarketable in many areas of the world. GMO foods are already unaccepted in Japan and as Americans become more aware of the untested safety aspects and the absence of any labeling requirement for GMO foods, many will reject them also."

In 2004, the Coalition to Protect Hawai'i Coffee expanded to include farmers and processors statewide. At this point the state Department of Agriculture, UH and HARC decided to stop research on GMO coffee and not field test the plants at that time. The consensus on this issue within the conflicted coffee industry was historic. Considering how fast GMO contamination can spread, stopping GMO crops before they are released is the best way to prevent contamination of our heritage crops.

Efforts to genetically transform taro also created outcry amongst Native Hawaiians and taro farmers (see page 68). Pineapple was being genetically engineered. Banana was being transformed to be resistant to bunchy top virus. A bio-pharmaceutical sugarcane was field-tested in 2005 in a secret location.

In 2008, Hawai'i County passed a law banning the research on, field-trialing of, or planting of GMO coffee and taro for 10 years. In 2009, Maui County banned GMO taro. Since that time, Hawai'i based researchers have gotten the message that our specialty crop industries don't want GMOs. These growers can't risk what the papaya farmers went through with the GMO contamination and market loss.

Melanie Bondera is an organic farmer in Kona who became concerned with GMOs in Hawai'i when she realized they threaten her family's livelihood and her children's health. She was a co-founder and director of Hawai'i GEAN and Hawai'i SEED. Melanie has worked to bring to light the extensive GMO Papaya contamination, and with the Hawai'i coffee industry in order to prevent GMO coffee from being field tested. She develops cooperatives around the state from the Laulima Center in order to rebuild the food system.

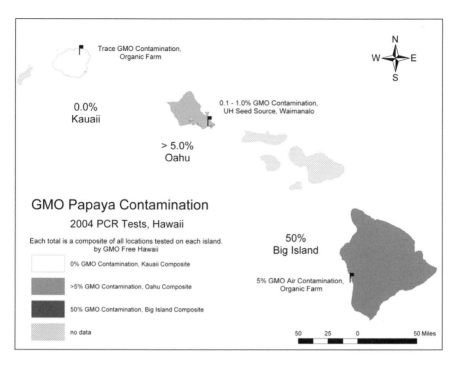

Trace GMO Contamination,
Organic Farm

N
W ✦ E
S

0.0%
Kauaii

0.1 - 1.0% GMO Contamination,
UH Seed Source, Waimanalo

> 5.0%
Oahu

GMO Papaya Contamination
2004 PCR Tests, Hawaii

Each total is a composite of all locations tested on each island.
by GMO Free Hawaii

0% GMO Contamination, Kauaii Composite

>5% GMO Contamination, Oahu Composite

50% GMO Contamination, Big Island Composite

no data

50%
Big Island

5% GMO Air Contamination,
Organic Farm

50   25   0   50 Miles

Unintended Consequences?
A Look at Potential Impact on Farmers

Luke Anderson

While some in Hawai'i's government, universities and communities tout biotechnology – and specifically genetic engineering of agricultural crops – as a potential boon to Hawai'i's economy, there are many who question whether embracing GMOs is a prudent, or even viable, approach. Within the context of Hawai'i's agricultural scene, it is important that we closely examine the ways in which local farmers could be negatively affected.

If crops become contaminated by DNA from GMOs, farmers could suffer losses in sales and in the public trust of the purity of crops and seeds produced in Hawai'i. Farmers would also lose the economic advantage in international and local markets of guaranteed GMO-free produce and the people of these islands would lose the right to buy locally grown produce that was free of contamination by DNA from genetically engineered crops.

How could GMO contamination happen?

- **Seed:** people buy unlabeled GMO foods in the market and plant them unknowingly (e.g. papaya, corn).
- **Cross-pollination:** wind or insects can carry pollen over large distances. (Genetically engineered corn can contaminate corn being grown on farms or in backyard gardens)
- **Animals:** genetically engineered seed can be picked up by birds, pigs, goats and other animals and deposited at another location
- **Mechanical:** through farm equipment, commingling during processing and storage, or during transport.
- **Through the passing of DNA** from plant material into the soil where it can be transferred to microorganisms.

Has GMO contamination already been experienced by farmers in Hawai'i?

Farmers growing genetically engineered papayas in Hawai'i have already experienced this problem – markets in Japan and Korea have refused to accept our genetically engineered papayas, although Japan accepted the importation of GMO papayas in 2012 provided they are labeled as such.

There is also evidence that people in Hawai'i have been unwittingly planting genetically engineered papayas in their backyard gardens and on their farms. Hawai'i SEED sent samples of papaya seed from organic farms, backyard gardens and wild trees to Genetic ID, one of the world's leading independent scientific laboratories for genetic contamination testing. The results revealed widespread contamination on Hawai'i Island. Contamination was also found in one variety of non-genetically engineered seeds being sold commercially by the University of Hawai'i (UH). A number of organic growers decided to chop their papaya trees down after the contamination was discovered (see "Papaya and Coffee," page 47).

"These tests indicate that some of UH's non-GMO seed stock is contaminated, and so there can be no doubt that the University must take immediate action to protect farmers, consumers and the environment," said Mark Query of Hawai'i SEED. "Papaya contamination is a case-study in the threat that GMO contamination presents to local agriculture. It is now obvious that coexistence of traditional and GMO crops is impossible. Coexistence means contamination."

What happens if an organic farm gets contaminated?

To be sold or labeled as organic, food has to be grown and processed without the use of genetic engineering. Evidence from recent years shows that contamination from genetically engineered crops is already causing serious problems for organic farms. It is affecting the value of farm produce and costing some farmers tens of thousands of dollars.[1] Organic buyers demand that organic food crops are free from genetic contamination, which can happen through cross-pollination, and these consumers will refuse to purchase organic produce if it has been affected in this way.[2]

The U.S. Department of Agriculture (USDA) organic standards are somewhat ambiguous about "accidental contamination." Some farmers and organic certifiers have been told by the USDA that no one should lose organic certification as a result of accidental GMO contamination. But the rules are clear that if an organic certifier has any reason to believe that GMO contamination may have happened on an organic farm, testing can be required.[3] If this testing shows that there has been GMO contamination, the farmer would lose organic certification. According to Richard H. Matthews of the USDA National Organic Program (NOP), "what happens to the farmer's land when GMO seeds are planted, knowingly or unknowingly? The answer to that is the land must go through a new three-year conversion."[4]

Farmers have also been told by NOP representatives that the NOP would never decertify a farmer for an accidental planting of a GMO crop, indicating that there is some confusion regarding this issue at the NOP. In order for the discriminating consumer to have faith in the organic system, farmers are asking that the NOP clarify and tighten its regulations.

Many organic farmers are facing increased costs and work due to measures they are taking to prevent contamination. These measures include increasing the distances between crops to try to prevent cross-pollination, adjusting timing of planting, altering cropping patterns or crops produced, changing cropping locations, careful consideration of seed sources, and talking with neighbors.

Who pays if a farmer's crop becomes contaminated?

Genetic engineering corporations work hard to avoid safety testing and labeling of GMOs by asserting that they are essentially the same as foods produced by any other breeding method. However, because the opposite stance also suits the industry, it freely describes GMOs as being radically different so that new inventions that can be patented.

Monsanto, the corporation responsible for most of the world's genetically engineered crops, controls these patents by forcing farmers who buy genetically engineered seeds to sign a "technology agreement." This agreement allows Monsanto to conduct investigations on the farmer's land and binds the farmer to Monsanto's oversight for multiple years. It also exposes farmers to huge financial liability.

Farmers have been found technically liable for infringements of Monsanto's patents even when the farmers' fields were contaminated by pollen or seed from someone else's genetically engineered crop or when genetically engineered seed from a previous year's crop sprouted in fields planted with non-genetically engineered varieties the following year. By 2004 Monsanto had filed 90 lawsuits against farmers in the United States. For cases with recorded judgments, farmers ended up having to pay Monsanto an average of $412,259.[5]

"Instead of supporting untested technologies like genetic engineering," says Dr. Héctor Valenzuela of UH Manoa's Department of Plant and Environmental Protection Sciences, "the University of Hawai'i should redirect their resources to focus on researching and promoting workable, non-GMO solutions to local agricultural problems. Hawai'i farmers need agricultural advances that can protect their farms and our state's agricultural economy over the long run."

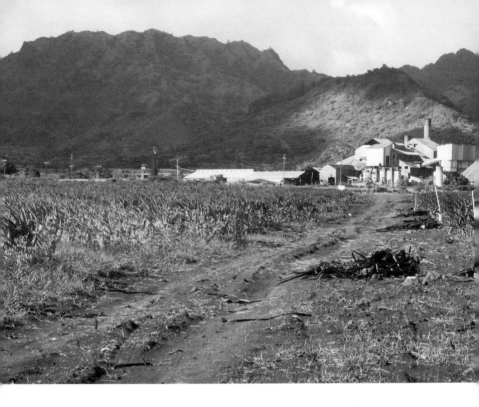

From Plantations to GMOs
The Struggle for the Farming Future of West Kaua'i

Phoebe Eng

> *In 'olelo Hawai'i, the mother tongue of these islands, "wai" is*
> *water, "waiwai" means values or wealth, and "kānāwai" is*
> *the law. It is no coincidence that, in an island community like*
> *ours, both wealth and the law were, and continue to be, defined*
> *by fresh water.*

> —From *Ola I Ka Wai: A Legal Primer for Water Use and Land*
> *Management in Hawai'i*[1]

The history of land and power in Hawai'i is tied to water. By understanding who controls the flow and direction of our islands' waters, we can also understand who determines the fate of *Hawai'i nei*, its agricultural destiny and its people.

The ongoing story of water and its connection to power in Hawai'i is well demonstrated in Kaua'i. Here, on this island's West Side – the leeward, drier side of Kaua'i – a battle for control of water is taking shape. Hydropower project sponsors, GMO companies, Hawaiian taro farmers with *lo'i* on Kuleana[2] Lands, native Hawaiian Home Lands beneficiaries, and state agencies like the Hawai'i Department of Agriculture and Hawai'i Department of Land and Natural Resources (DLNR) are now negotiating for control and attempting to clarify their rights with regard to west Kaua'i water.

At the heart of this struggle is the future development of the West Side, the fate of the GMO industry on Kaua'i, and the viability of a new era of local, sustainable agriculture in this region.

A Short History of Water on West Kaua'i

The modern history of water use on the West Side starts in the late 1870s, when sugar growing replaced the smaller scale rice fields and *lo'i* cultivated by Chinese and Hawaiian farmers.[3]

On the West Side, Kekaha Sugar Company and then American Factors (Amfac/JMB) developed the Koke'e and Kekaha Ditch systems that diverted large amounts of water from intakes in the upland swamps and forests to sugarcane lands that extend from Waimea to Mana.[4] Also included in the plantation water and irrigation systems were a series of reservoirs that collected and stored water, along with groundwater wells that brought potable water to plantation workers.

Enter the Agribusiness Development Corporation

The Hawai'i sugar market decline of the late 1990s, and the abrupt exit of the West Side plantations shortly thereafter, had huge economic implications for the area.[5] Abandoned sugarcane lands reverted back to the state, to the DLNR, and in 1994, the State Legislature created a new state agency, the Agribusiness Development Corporation (ADC) within the Department of Agriculture to manage the transition of those lands. ADC is charged with transitioning the monocrop operations of the former plantations into new diversified agriculture enterprises, and managing former sugarcane lands toward that overall goal.[6]

The ADC, however, is not an ordinary public agency. It is granted powers that enable it to contract with private sector partners more quickly than other public sector agencies.[7] ADC formally assumed management responsibility of approximately 12,500 acres of Kekaha agricultural lands in late 2003 under Executive Order No. 4007.[8] From that acreage, 7,750 acres are considered to be Kekaha's most productive lands, and approximately 5,300 acres (the fertile *makai* acres on the coastal Kekaha-Mana plain) have since been given, through a restrictive use easement, to the Pacific Missile Range Facility, for a low intensity agricultural buffer zone.[9] This land giveaway by the state was hotly contested by native Hawaiian leaders and community members, yet unanimously passed by the Board of Land and Natural Resources (BLNR). The motion to pass was made by Lynn McCrory, then a BLNR member and currently co-owner of Kekaha Sugar Mill.[10] Those restrictive use acres are currently leased to GMO companies.[11]

GMO Moves In

GMO companies became the true controllers of West Side land and water in 2007. In that year, ADC gave the exclusive license to use, manage, operate, maintain and control the infrastructure of the west Kaua'i former sugar cane lands to a private entity called Kekaha Agriculture Association.[12] This broad control includes management of the Koke'e and Kekaha ditch systems and the control and taking of its flows. For its services, KAA receives sizeable annual management fees and project fees funded with taxpayer dollars, and perhaps indirectly through government subsidies. In 2009 for example, KAA received at least one project fee of $581,250 to relocate electrical equipment from the Kekaha Sugar Mill.[13]

KAA often describes itself as a "farmers cooperative" of leaseholders of the west Kaua'i state-owned lands. However, it is currently run and primarily financed by its largest corporate members, which to date include the GMO companies Pioneer Hi-Bred International (a division of the chemical company giant, DuPont), Syngenta (the Swiss chemical company that created the widespread herbicide Atrazine), and BASF (a transnational chemical company headquartered in Germany).[14]

In many ways, KAA has merely recreated the plantation system in its "top down" approach to land and water management. As with plantations, the ultimate decision makers of GMO companies are far away from the communities directly impacted by their companies' environmental practices.[15]

No publicly promoted, diversified agriculture training to Kaua'i's aspiring farmer population has been noticeably forthcoming from KAA, and no real progress has yet been made on West Side agricultural lands in developing what Kaua'i's people say they want: an island that can be "food secure" even in times of emergency; and produce affordable, healthy and nutritious fresh food locally among small family-owned farms that use sustainable agricultural practices.

ADC, in choosing the GMO industry-dominant KAA as its West Side land manager, has shortchanged its fiduciary duty to transition the West Side's former sugarcane lands into diversified agriculture. In doing so, the state also forgoes the opportunity to explore new land and water management practices that could transform west Kaua'i into an important center for sustainable, diversified agriculture, and revitalize West Side local economies through smaller-scale, locally-owned farming enterprises.

Hydropower Interests

In a new twist on the old plantation model, KAA is also advancing the privatization of the West Side's water to produce hydropower. A hydropower developer, Pacific Light and Power (PLP), incorporated under Delaware law, is a new licensee of West Side *mauka* land, currently leasing ADC land at $15 per acre annually, and is a member of KAA.[16]

As well-meaning as their alternative energy plans may be, PLP (through its wholly-owned subsidiary Konohiki Hydro Power) intends to develop hydropower infrastructure that will use the water flows of the Koke'e and Kekaha ditches, and burn guinea grass from their leased lands to create power exclusively for the needs of the KAA private sector members. According to PLP, public funds may be used to pay for this project, even though the benefits will inure to the private sector.[17] PLP proposes to sell excess power to Kaua'i's public utility, Kaua'i Island Utility Company (KIUC), a rural cooperative that is owned by the people of Kaua'i.[18] This energy sale back to the people would be an additional income source for the private sector.

Possible Violations of the "Public Trust" Doctrine

When private sector interests are the primary beneficiaries of state-owned natural resources, such as our water and our fertile soil, the public trust benefits of Kaua'i's resources are no longer guaranteed.

When non-transparent, plantation-style management practices continue to determine West Side water and land use, our communities cannot advance toward more sustainable agricultural practices that could produce a higher, healthier quality of life for Kaua'i's taxpaying residents.

KAA's management approach has been to put Kaua'i's rich soil, water and abundant sunshine largely into the service of producing non-edible test crops for GMO companies. The pesticide and herbicide practices of GMO tenants damage our soil over the long term, reducing it to a lifeless growing medium.[19] Open air GMO chemical spraying is affecting the health of West Side children and families, resulting in increased health care costs that are borne by taxpayers, insurance companies and private citizens.[20] The green waste generated in these test fields may also be plowed back into our soil or deposited into our landfills due to lack of meaningful regulation. Grubbing[21] violations of GMO companies may have adversely affected West Side estuary ecosystems and coral reefs.[22]

Additionally, under KAA management, Kekaha and Koke'e Ditch systems continue to divert water from the Waimea River, possibly limiting the habitat and swimming range of native Hawaiian fish species such as 'o'opu.[23] Decreased river flows may also concentrate bacteria and pollutants into smaller amounts of water downstream, which could explain why, according to local accounts, West Side children are frequently falling ill after swimming in the river. Perhaps due to less water flow from upriver, silt builds up at the mouth of the Waimea River, resulting a higher, drier bed at the river mouth, and preventing a healthy, fresh water flow from *mauka* to *makai*.[24]

To add insult to injury, much of West Side ditch water, which was historically needed to irrigate sugarcane, is now siphoned away from the lowlands through a series of pumps, in order to keep the *makai* GMO fields from becoming too wet for the GMO companies' test crops (predominantly corn). The result is ironic: KAA currently generates power from its privately-run *mauka* powerhouses to divert the unwanted water away from its own land.[25] This diversion will likely continue unless and until such time as KAA may want the excess water for its hydropower businesses currently in development.[26]

Hawaiian Water Law and the "Public Trust" Doctrine

Hawai'i has some of the strongest water and stream flow protection standards in the nation, and clearly states that "public trust" water uses, and specifically native Hawaiian uses, have the priority claim to water in our state. Hawai'i water law could therefore be critical in determining the long term viability of the GMO industry in west Kaua'i.

Among the key laws and concepts that inform the "public trust" doctrine, perhaps one of the most fundamental, in *Article 11, Sec 1* of the *Hawai'i*

Constitution, maintains that "all public natural resources are held in trust by the State for the benefit of the people."[27]

Kuleana,[28] appurtenant[29] and traditional native Hawaiian customary rights, as well as riparian rights[30] are expressly protected under the public trust doctrine.[31] Public trust uses have priority over private commercial uses, which do not enjoy the same protection. The law dictates that "any balancing between public and private purposes must begin with a presumption in favor of public use, access, and enjoyment."[32] Stream diversions that propose to use water for private commercial gain have the burden of justifying these uses against protected public rights to the water. Kuleana rights have a priority over "off-stream" uses and cannot be lost, even if they are not currently utilized.[33]

The Water Code also gives priority protection to "appurtenant rights"[34] and traditional customary rights such as cultivating kalo and gathering various natural resources for subsistence, cultural, and religious purposes, such as *hihiwai*, *opae*, *'o'opu*, *limu*, thatch, ti leaf, *aho* cord, and medicinal plants.[35]

If KAA's management of the water infrastructure has effectively denied or limited the ability of native Hawaiians or the Hawaiian people to exercise any of these public trust purposes, management and control of water by KAA runs afoul of these legal principles.

What is also clear is that the proactive exercise of native Hawaiian rights to West Side water, supported by strong policies that defend established water law, can change the long-term direction of West Side agriculture and regional economic development.

The West Side Vision

As Kaua'i voters become more aware of the importance of water rights in determining the future of our island, we can begin to explore alternatives that serve the public trust and encourage our elected officials to do the same.

Kaua'i's West Side community is home to some of the poorest families on the island today, and historically its concerns have largely been ignored by state and county government. But in their emerging courage to speak up, through core values that prioritize health, cultural wisdom, community, and *malama 'aina*, the West Side can change the course of its destiny. Its residents can then identify the most appropriate and *pono* collaborators for transitioning away from plantation-based, paternalistic ways of doing business. Through that transition, the West Side can become a world-class destination and model for sustainable regional development.

Here is a picture of a better West Side future: restoring the ditch flows back into the river could allow for the re-introduction of *lo'i* and sustainable *ahupua'a* systems that nurture larger populations of *'o'opu* and other native species. A new generation of farmers might learn to grow food by working with the principles of small-scale, locally-based sustainable agriculture, aquaculture, and pastoral practices. New locally-owned businesses based on value-added agricultural products could revitalize the regional economies of Kekaha and Waimea. Young West Siders would have a broader range of life choices and opportunities.

With water flowing through the *mauka* home lands above Kekaha at Pu'u Opae, training of native Hawaiian homesteaders in new, biodynamic farming practices could fulfill the promise of the Hawaiian Homes Act. New groups, such as Ka Piko o Waimea, which intends to revitalize Waimea Valley's taro culture and the Kekaha Community Garden that teaches residents how to farm nutritious foods, could thrive.

Water law may be the catalyst that creates a tipping point for that vision. Restoring instream flows, putting West Side waters back into the river, developing strong policies that truly honor the "public trust," and re-establishing the *'ahupua'a*[36] and *kuleana* relationship between land, water, and the people, could be the West Side's greatest gift to the world.

Mahalo nui loa to EarthJustice for its longtime dedication to the protection of water rights for the people of Hawai'i.

Phoebe Eng is a community advocate and has been an advisor to several social and environmental justice organizations and national foundations. A former attorney, Eng believes strongly that "knowledge is power." She currently focuses on providing Hawaiian communities with the facts they do not have – but often need – to understand their historical, political, and economic context and fight effectively for change.

A Vision for Sustainable Agriculture
Our Historic Food Sovereignty Can Be Restored

Nancy Redfeather and Melanie Bondera

The planters of Old Hawai'i had a vision and knowledge of ecological, sustainable agriculture. Verdant farms and gardens stretching *mauka* to *makai* formed the *ahupua'a* system that produced enough food for large populations on all islands. Today we think of "ecological" as meaning that which works in harmony with Nature, and "sustainable" as a system that will continue to produce over many generations without degrading the soil upon which agriculture rests. This is the kind of agriculture we need for Hawai'i's future.

After the arrival of Captain Cook, successive waves of plantation agriculture dominated Hawai'i's landscape. When the plantation system finally crashed, everyone began to talk of diversified agriculture. This new system would replace the huge mono-crops of pineapple and sugar that were owned by a few companies, which paid low wages to workers and often polluted soils with pesticides and agro-chemicals, with a more community-friendly model. The vision of many small farms owned by the people, growing diverse crops with multiple markets, began to expand. This type of system creates food security and food sovereignty, which is important for our remote island chain.

But in the early 1990s Governor Ben Cayetano and our agricultural decision makers had a different plan in mind. Their blueprint would replace plantation agriculture with genetically engineered agriculture. Corporations genetically engineering agricultural crops were invited to move here and were given sufficient financial incentives to keep them here (see "GMOs in Hawai'i – the Big Picture," page 25). Now 20 years later, Hawai'i is the center for open air field testing of experimental GMO crops and corn seed development of GMO feed corn destined for United States farms. Hawai'i taxpayers have subsidized this industry heavily – and what have been the benefits? Seed crops are exported and profits flow to corporations outside Hawai'i. The open experimental field trials are difficult to regulate and have

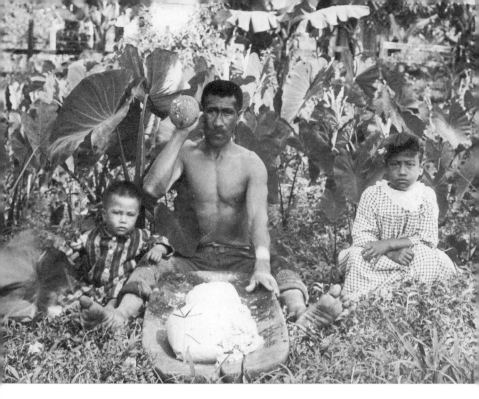

unknown effects on our ʻāina, ecosystems, and health of the community. Our fragile environment, the intricate balance of which we barely understand, is in danger of being polluted by living reproducing organisms that cannot be contained. It is now commonly known that once a genetically engineered agricultural crop is planted in a geographical region, it is only a matter of time before conventional and organic farmers will experience genetic contamination of their crops. We have traded this real consequence for a handful of low-wage jobs.

We should remind ourselves that from the moment that settlers first landed in the Hawaiian islands until the 1960s we were food self-sufficient. Today, we import over 85 percent of our food. Our dependence on oil to transport our food across longer and longer distances, and on oil-based fertilizers that fuel industrial agriculture, is increasingly cost prohibitive. What will replace this fossil-fuel dependent, industrial model that has degraded soils and farming communities worldwide?

There is another vision. Land reform at the state and county level can create affordable opportunities for interested farmers to live and farm long-term on a piece of land. We need to keep our best agricultural lands zoned for agriculture and continue to develop water infrastructure. Our institutions can develop educational programs that actually train young people and mid-career changers to farm in the tropics. Counties can work with farmers to recycle the communities' organic waste, which will increase soil health and farm profitability. The Cooperative Extension Services can offer non-toxic solutions to pests and disease and assist communities with knowledge for developing community and home gardens. The University of Hawai'i can develop open-pollinated seed varieties of both fruits and vegetables adapted to our tropical environment. Our Rural Economic Development boards can support direct marketing of agricultural products such as farmers markets and CSAs (community supported agriculture). Farmers in the community can form cooperative businesses to market wholesale. Schools can purchase fresh produce from local farms. Supermarkets can buy local produce, and restaurants can feature fresh foods from area farms for the visitor and local alike.

Working together, these programs form a new vision of agriculture, a vision that is gathering interest locally and already growing in many areas of the United States and elsewhere in the world. Perhaps the most compelling aspect of the sustainable food movement is how quickly a community can create a local food economy. It doesn't take global agreements and it doesn't require new legislation. Each time we buy food from a local farmer who grows in ways that respect the land, we are voting for a safer, economically vibrant and more delicious food system and way of life in Hawai'i.

We have incredible potential here with our vigorous year-round growing environment. We can grow valuable high-end tropical fruits, nuts, vegetables and flowers for specialty markets. We can feed our families and our communities. We can focus on diversified niche markets and value-added products. We can assist our farmers to procure small grants for processing machinery and development of business plans. We can be the center of tropical agricultural research and program application for farmers in the tropical countries of the world!

Instead of using our land as a laboratory, we can connect to the ancient sustainable and profitable farming systems that have been practiced here in Hawai'i and on planet Earth for 10,000 years. We can demand that our institutions be responsive and responsible to our communities and land, rebalancing our farming systems in the ecological/sustainable ways of the future.

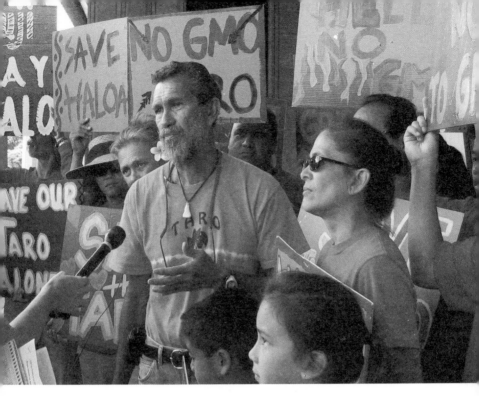

Engaging the Grassroots
"Uncle" Walter Ritte Takes on GMOs

Catherine Mariko Black

Walter Ritte is already a legendary name in Hawaiian activism and the Aloha 'Āina movement. A veteran of many watershed issues in Hawaiian rights – including the historic battle to reclaim Kaho'olawe, the State Constitutional Convention of 1978 and the creation of the Office of Hawaiian Affairs – he has also led countless efforts to preserve his native Moloka'i island's agricultural and traditional subsistence-based lifestyle.

In recent years, these values have led to Ritte's involvement in the debate around GMOs. As a cultural activist and community leader, Ritte has been one of the most visible individuals to bring the issue down to the grassroots and engage people – Hawaiians and non-Hawaiians – on a personal level in the discussion.

Ritte's own commitment was ignited by the University of Hawai'i's

(UH) research efforts to genetically engineer and patent taro (see "The Fight Over Hāloa," page 68). When the notion of modifying taro in a laboratory and putting a stamp of intellectual property on it came to light, it created a public outcry and Ritte voiced the concern of many Hawaiians about the project's ethical and spiritual ramifications.

"It felt like we were being violated by the scientific community, like our privacy was being invaded. And this is because, for the Hawaiian community, taro is not just a plant – it's a family member, it's our common ancestor Hāloa. Our reaction was: *How dare you tamper with and patent a family member without our permission?*"

Over the past few decades, taro has assumed increasing importance as a symbol of Hawaiian cultural identity, food sovereignty and an integrated model of sustainable resource conservation for the islands. People were already exploring taro as it related to protecting land and water resources and instilling a new environmental ethic, so when the UH patenting issue came up, it struck a deep chord. "When the discussion about GMO involved Hāloa, it took on a traditional resonance and that's what brought the Hawaiian community in," remembers Ritte.

In addition, the replacement of Moloka'i Ranch by Monsanto as the island's largest employer has brought the issue home for Ritte in a very concrete way. "Monsanto came in the middle of the night, and on Moloka'i that's hard to do because we are a small community where everyone knows when someone new arrives on island." Several years after Monsanto had bought existing seed companies like Hawaiian Research for their GMO field testing, it became clear that the quiet but powerful new neighbor was not just another farming operation.

Ritte believes that on an island with such a deeply ingrained agricultural identity, GMO companies and their practices are increasingly alarming. "They're buying up our Ag water and using these unsustainable growing methods like plowing the fields four times a year, which leaves the soil bare. Today, people on Moloka'i are driving through a dust bowl, and there are probably chemicals in that dust, which then rise into the clouds and fall back into the water table."

Despite all this, GMO continues to be an issue of "quiet resistance" on Moloka'i. As in other parts of Hawai'i, conflicts involving big business often threaten the social fabric of small communities, where the lack of economic opportunity inevitably means that families are divided or pitted against each other. Ritte says that waging an all-out war against GMO on

Moloka'i would not only be logistically difficult, but emotionally draining. Instead, he is focusing his energies on raising awareness and influencing the political and decision-making on O'ahu.

Ritte helped form the Label It Hawai'i coalition, which is organizing in support of state legislation to require the commercial labeling of genetically modified foods. "We feel that education is the best place to start when it comes to GMO," he says. "Taro was a narrower issue – that was about Hāloa – but now it's much bigger. For Hawaiians, the focus has expanded to look at what these GMO companies are doing to the land. To us, Hāloa represents all of our environmental resources and our ability to take care of them, by recognizing that the 'āina is what feeds us and keeps us alive. The GMO issue now is not just about taro, it's about Aloha 'Āina."

Although not everyone can engage with the more scientific or environmental nuances of the GMO debate, Ritte distills it into material that everyday people can identify with. "Labeling affects not only Hawaiians, but all of us. For anyone who cares about the health of their families, this is a personal question that involves mothers and fathers." He emphasizes that GMO labeling is less about political ideology or cultural background, and more about people's right to know what they are consuming and feeding their children.

With the patience of an old-timer who has waged many David-and-Goliath battles, Ritte adds, "We're starting from zero, but the good thing about starting from zero is that there's nowhere to go but up."

Walter Ritte is a recognized Hawaiian activist whose long political and grassroots organizing career includes many milestones in the movement for Hawaiian cultural, political and environmental rights. As an "Aloha 'Āina" warrior, his accomplishments include protecting traditional access rights on his home island of Moloka'i; the occupation of Kaho'olawe that resulted in a halt to U.S. Navy's use of the island as a bombing target and its return to the State of Hawai'i; the creation of the Office of Hawaiian Affairs, of which he was a founding board member; and a number of initiatives to preserve traditional cultural and environmental resources on Moloka'i, including the rebuilding of ancient fishponds and the protection of the island's South Shore from development. He is on the Board of Directors of Hawai'i SEED.

The Fight Over Hāloa

In 2002, the University of Hawai'i (UH) patented three varieties of hybridized (non-genetically engineered) taro. These were descendants of the Hawaiian-Polynesian taro group, "Lehua." This patenting required farmers wishing to purchase huli, or breeding stock, to sign a licensing agreement with UH. The licensing agreement stated that "UH owns the taro cultivar..." It prohibited farmers from selling or breeding the patented plants, and required the payment of a royalty to the University. In 2003, UH, in conjunction with the Hawai'i Agriculture Research Center (HARC), began genetic engineering of three varieties of taro. They experimented with inserting rice, wheat and grapevine genes into the Chinese (Bunlong), Hawaiian (Maui Lehua) and Samoan (Niue) taro and were successful with the Bunlong variety. But when Hawaiians, taro farmers and other concerned citizens learned about what was happening, they put up a formidable resistance.

Walter Ritte was one of the most visible members of the Hawaiian community to lead protests on the issue. "We called it the 'Mana Mahele' because we felt that what was happening to Hāloa was the same thing that had happened to our lands [in the Great Mahele of 1848]," says Ritte. "The scientists were going to modify, patent and own Hāloa, an ancestor and family member of the Hawaiian people. They weren't satisfied with just taking our land; now they wanted to take our *mana*, or spirit, too." Among other actions, Ritte helped to organize a high-profile protest on May 18, 2006, in which UH students chained the doors to a Board of Regents meeting at the UH John H. Burns School of Medicine.

On June 16th, 2006 UH dropped its patents on the three varieties of taro.

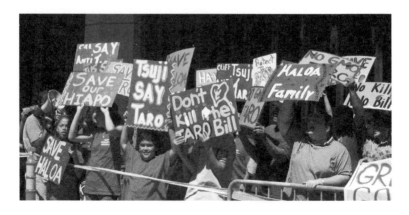

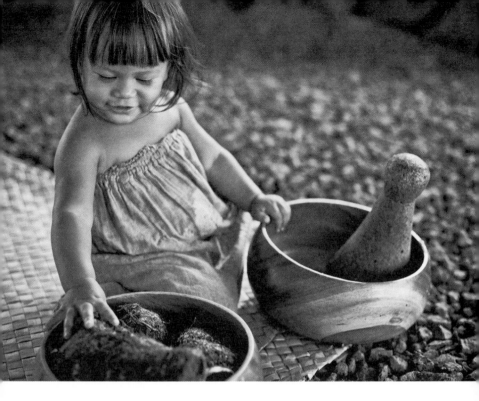

Activating your 'Umeke Kūmau
The Story Behind Legalizing Pa'i 'Ai

Daniel Anthony

The story I want to share with you is about conflicting lifestyles, cultures and mentalities. For me and others like me, the GMO issue is what originally spurred a new generation of Hawaiians to look at taro farming as a potential lifestyle reality. It was the year 2006 and there was uproar in the community over the University of Hawai'i's efforts to patent genetically engineered taro. At the time, I was a sales executive working for a natural stone company. I had also just started going to the Waiahole Mauka Lo'i to pull taro, which I would pound into *pa'i 'ai* (hand-pounded taro before being diluted into poi) to eat at home.

I remember the opening of the 2008 Legislative Session, when there was a massive rally and camp-out accompanied by taro pounding or *ku'i 'ai* at the State Capitol and 'Iolani Palace. At this event I spoke with many

kupuna, and they all told me the same thing: "Hāloa needs more farmers."
I took this message to heart and began researching taro farming, but the
more I researched, the more disheartened I became. The farm gate price of
taro was sixty cents per pound, which meant that to gross 100,000 dollars
annually I would need to farm almost 160,000 pounds per year! On top of
that, there were the stories I'd heard about the loss of land and water, family
conflicts, the development of *lo'i kalo* (taro patches) for luxury homes, hotels
and shopping centers … it all seemed so backward, and was only making me
angry at the world. I was starting to see that the current system is merely
set up for minimum wage laborers, not real taro farmers.

A Road to Change

This is when I decided that I would have to change the taro industry itself
if I wanted a future in it. So I reverse engineered the process, starting from
the price that I would need to sell taro at in order to make a decent living.
Two dollars per pound is the farm gate price I came up with that would
make it worthwhile for me to farm high quality, chemical and fertilizer-free
taro. Although it is harder to cultivate taro organically, I was lucky enough
to grow up in an environment that taught me the importance of clean
farming. Today, when I eat fresh taro, I can actually taste whether there's
chemical fertilizer in it, and I can see the effects of Roundup, which shows
up as little brown pimples on the corm.

So I started to pay the taro farmers I knew two dollars per pound,
and I pounded that taro with a traditional board (*papa ku'i 'ai*) and stone
(*pohaku ku'i 'ai*) to promote native Hawaiian art. Suddenly there was an
influx of invitations to pound taro at events. At around this time I attended
Papakū Makawalu, a cultural practitioner workshop hosted by the Kanaka'ole
family on the Big Island. It was here that I publicly announced that I was
challenging myself to pound 10,000 pounds of taro. In 2009 I accepted
every single event invitation, farmer's market and other opportunity that
would help me to reach that goal.

Although it might have seemed crazy at first, what I learned through
that challenge is that not all taro is created equal. We bought around 20,000
pounds of taro that year, and we realized that some taro actually *is* worth
only sixty cents a pound – even less to us – because we couldn't turn it into
good pa'i 'ai (for which you need corms with high levels of starch, rather
than sugar). So to continue paying two dollars per pound, we began to
demand that quality from our farmers. Some of them got it and started

to cater to us by pulling their taro early, before its sugar content rises. On the flip side, these farmers began to use our taro purchases to leverage the poi companies to raise their buying price of taro and these poi companies were getting mad.

In September of 2009 we officially launched Mana Ai as a business. In October a photo of us pounding taro at the Ward Avenue Farmer's Market appeared in the Honolulu Advertiser. We had been pounding under a cultural and artistic premise before, but now we were pounding to sell. The following week the Department Of Health (DOH) went to the market, but we weren't there. Then they went to Haili's Hawaiian Foods, where we were scheduled to pound, and threatened to revoke their permit if our pa'i 'ai was sold there, which Aunty Rachel had to tell me with tears in her eyes when I showed up with forty pounds of taro.

We called the DOH and they told us that it was illegal to pound poi and serve it off the board because this process didn't adhere to health and safety regulations. We said, "Great, because we're pounding pa'i 'ai not poi," but they said, "Don't be silly" and threatened to fine us one thousand dollars a day for violations. KITV4 News contacted me, the Honolulu Weekly wrote an article and some Office of Hawaiian Affairs (OHA) attorneys went down to the DOH to talk. The DOH stood firm, saying that even in a certified kitchen we would not be able to make pa'i 'ai legally with our traditional wood and porous stone utensils, since these materials did not meet the FDA guidelines for sanitary food preparation. The Hale'iwa Taro Festival in November 2009 was the last time we sold pa'i 'ai openly until 2011.

Outside the Law

The DOH's decision created a conflict within our own business, and my best friend, with whom I had started Mana Ai, left to remove himself from liability. When he asked what I was going to do, I said I would inspire a law student at UH and we would change the regulations. Even my best friend told me I was stupid and it was a waste of time. But sure enough, in December of 2009 I linked up with Amy Brinker, who had read the articles about us, and was interested in writing her final law school paper on legalizing pa'i 'ai. At this time, we had gone "black market" with our product. It was just like selling pot. People would pull up to my house at all hours of the day or night, I would run out with a bag and they would pass me money.

But our focus was also changing. We knew that acting alone there was no way to influence the DOH. We also knew that feeding people hand-pounded paʻi ʻai was absolutely the right thing to do, and that we needed to create more awareness in the community so that other people could reach the same conclusion. So we began teaching people to make their own paʻi ʻai. The DOH could regulate us selling paʻi ʻai but they couldn't regulate people making their own for personal consumption. That year became all about community outreach, and at the end of 2010 we realized that we had sat down and pounded taro with 3,000 people. We had also identified twelve simple workshops for traditional poi-making proficiency.

That year at the La Hoʻi Hoʻi ʻEa Sovereignty Restoration event, we invited Amy Brinker to come down and talk about the paper that she had just finished writing. We also asked Uncle Earl Kawaʻa, an educator at Kamehameha Schools, to come down and do a board-making workshop with the traditional Hawaiian adze. These two met: the kupuna and the law student, and they began to work together.

In November of 2010 we participated in the Haleʻiwa Taro Festival again, and the festival's promotional material said that our paʻi ʻai was featured on the menu at Ed Kenney's Downtown restaurant. The following week, the DOH raided Downtown and actually stood and watched as restaurant staff throw away 20 pounds of paʻi ʻai. All throughout 2010, during our black market era, Ed Kenney had been carefully pairing paʻi ʻai with delicious meat, fish and poultry dishes, and serving it to the Honolulu community – including business people, lawmakers and politicians.

People never fight for what that they don't know, but once they have a taste for something and can no longer get it, they're willing to act. The paʻi ʻai story once more circulated in local media, and in December at a water cooler conversation in the OHA building, a trustee's aide asked a *lomi* practitioner, "What's up with this hand-pounding thing?" The practitioner said, "You should ask the guys that do it." So they called us up to sit down and talk about the issue.

Birth of a Political Movement

It was the first Thursday of December 2010, and OHA had brought together a group of taro farmers, taro pounders, educators and kupuna. Amy Brinker presented her Legalize Paʻi ʻai paper and at the end of the meeting, Uncle Earl Kawaʻa asked OHA, "So what are you going to do about this?" The OHA representative said, "I'm just here to listen, I can't make any promises." So Uncle Earl turned and faced the group of people to say, "ok gang, what are *we* going to do about it?" That moment was the birth of the Legalize

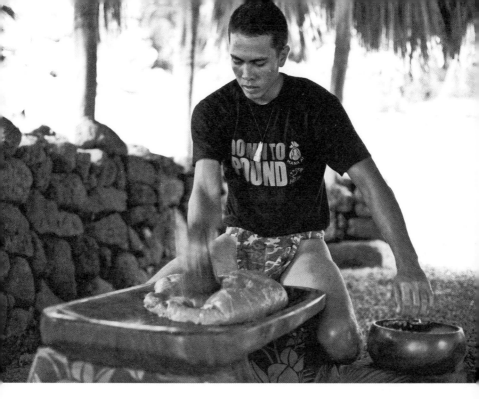

Pa'i 'ai 'Ohana. Of the twenty or so people that came to the first meeting, there were about ten strong ones that met every Thursday evening until May of 2011.

Legalizing pa'i 'ai boiled down to a small group of dedicated people who came together to strategize, research and implement lobbying practices that would fully engage the legislative system. For the first time, I personally saw how politics works. For example, I discovered that parties who may not be willing to talk to you directly will talk through the political process. I also realized that one of the benefits of working with politicians is that, at some point, they have to justify their positions by revealing their sources. And it's when the source is revealed that the community can begin to do its work. Without our politicians, we wouldn't have been able to identify the sources of opposition to our proposed "Poi Bill."

This was also the first time that I had seen Native Hawaiian institutions like OHA actively go out of their way to engage the parties that were in conflict with us to understand what the real problem was. OHA couldn't figure out how to bring those parties to the table, but they were able to identify what was bothering them: the real issue had more to do with a few key personalities and the fear of the costs of taro going up, than it had to do with legalizing paʻi ʻai or putting traditional foods back on the table. Then it was beautiful to see how the kupuna stepped in and did what the institutions couldn't do: negotiate and come to agreement.

Legalizing paʻi ʻai happened because everyone played their part: the activated individual (myself and others), the researcher (Amy Brinker), the educator (Earl Kawaʻa), the government institutions (DOH, State Senate and House of Representatives), the Hawaiian institutions (OHA) and above all, the kupuna. They were the ones who truly had our back. They also had the power that comes from ancestral relationships. Jerry Konanui, Earl Kawaʻa and Joe Tassell were the three kupuna without whom we would not have been able to do this. Our path led through many steps, but at every single turn the kupuna came in with very specific help. Though it seemed impossible at times, SB101 was approved on May 3, 2011.

But the real victory didn't happen then. The real victory lies in our ability to continue with this work. The victory is every board and every stone in each new ʻohana. Sustainability will never be real in Hawaiʻi if it's served on two scoops of Calrose white rice. We can build a new Hawaiʻi using taro on any level: we can buy it, we can learn about how to make food with it, we can learn how to make the traditional utensils and we can farm it. Every one of those actions supports our sustainability and sovereignty, which simply means not having to depend on someone else for your staple.

A staple is something that you eat three times a day. Taro is the staple food of Hawaiʻi and the staple is what holds the community and the culture together. If our staple is Hāloa, then Hāloa will bind us together. And if Hāloa can be a staple for our community once again, we are going to be held together very firmly.

Daniel Anthony is an advocate of traditional, hand-pounded poi and the deep-rooted cultural values that this Hawaiian staple food represents. In 2009, he co-founded Mana Ai, a local company that produces, distributes and promotes fresh, artisan poi and paʻi ʻai and has almost singlehandedly put these items on the contemporary map of new Island cuisine. Anthony was one of the driving forces behind the statewide movement to successfully pass legislation legalizing the public sale of hand-pounded poi. To further restore a culturally grounded vision of ecological and economic sustainability, Anthony and his wife co-founded the nonprofit organization Hui Aloha ʻĀina Momona in 2011. Driven by a vision of restoring ʻāina momona (abundant land) in Hawaiʻi, the organization engages the community in educational and cultural activities that include board-making workshops and founding school kuʻi clubs.

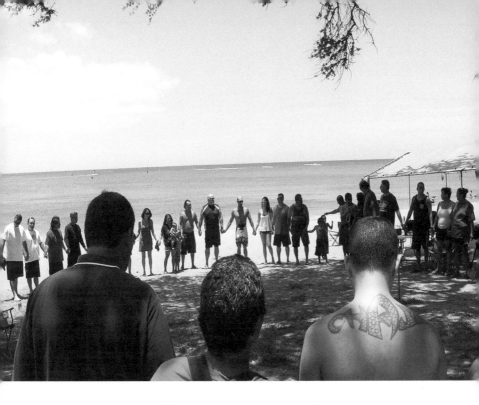

Hawaiian Perspectives
GMOs and Cultural Values

Mililani Trask

Genetic Manipulation of our Genealogy

The kalo is a primary staple food of Hawaiians and most other Polynesians, as well as Asians. As has been demonstrated by the Moloka'i Diet study and the Wai'anae diet study, kalo is a key to maintaining the health of Hawaiians who currently suffer from acute health problems including obesity, cancer, diabetes and heart conditions.

For Hawaiians, the research and experimentation undertaken by the University of Hawai'i and corporate entities on the kalo directly impacts their genealogy. This belief is based on Hawaiian oral histories and *oli* (genealogical chants) maintained by Hawaiians from time immemorial. As documented by Hawaiian ethno-botanist Isabella Abbot, according to these *oli*, the supreme god Kane "in the form of Wakea (a form associated with the earth) produced two sequential offspring: the first became the kalo (taro) plant, the second became Hāloa, the ancestor of man . . . Thus, in kinship terms, the taro is the elder brother and the senior branch of the family tree; mankind belongs to the junior branch, stemming from the younger brother." For Hawaiians, the kalo is literally part of their genealogy as well as the staff of life.

The Paoakalani Declaration

In October 2003, Hawaiian *kupuna* (elders), *kumu hula* (masters of hula), *makua* (adults), and '*opio* (youth) from all islands and all walks of life gathered on O'ahu to consider how best to perpetuate their culture and to protect their traditional knowledge. The meeting (referred to as Ka 'Aha Pono – the Righteous Gathering) concluded with the issuing of a collective statement entitled "The Paoakalani Declaration," which set forth the cultural perspective on many issues including GMOs, patenting of traditional knowledge and the commercial exploitation of Hawai'i's biodiversity.

For Hawai'i's indigenous peoples, the concepts underlying genetic manipulation of life forms is offensive and contrary to the cultural values of aloha 'āina (love for the land). Most importantly, Hawaiians view the current efforts of the University of Hawai'i, the United States, the State of Hawai'i, and pharmaceutical and transnational corporations to modify, patent and commercialize life forms as *hewa* (a wrongful act, an act of desecration of the sacred) which will bring imbalance and negativity into our lives and our environment. Hawai'i's indigenous peoples oppose GMOs because it is the *pono* (righteous) thing to do.

"We emphasize that the Kanaka Maoli worldview is governed by the cultural principles of pono, malama, 'āina and kuleana. Within this worldview, the Earth and her myriad life forms (biological diversity) are kinolau, the earthly body forms of the Akua. Every life form possesses living energy that sustains each other creating a familial, interdependent, reciprocal relationship between the Akua, the 'aina, and the kanaka in fine balance and harmony."

—From the Paokalani Declaration

Mililani B. Trask is a native Hawaiian attorney and an international indigenous legal expert. She has served as the Pacific Basin Expert to the United Nations Permanent Forum on Indigenous Issues and co-chaired the Sub-Committee on Indigenous Self-determination of the UN Intercessional Working Group on the Draft Declaration. Her 'ohana owns a farm in Hamakua which plants and markets organic 'awa, noni and neem.

How to Avoid Eating GE Foods

Jeffrey Smith and Hawai'i SEED

Until genetically engineered foods have been fully tested and proven safe by unbiased decision-makers, it would be wise to avoid eating them or serving them to your family. More and more people are choosing to eat organic and non-GMO foods (no product labeled "organic" may contain GE ingredients), and the following information will help you to identify which foods to avoid. Voting with your food dollars is one of the best ways to send industry and political decision-makers the message that consumers are concerned about the health consequences of eating these foods. For additional name brands of products containing GMO ingredients, consult the True Food Guide at www.truefoodnow.org/shoppers-guide/

Currently Commercialized GMO Crops in the U.S.
Soybean (93%), cotton (94%, cottonseed oil is often used in food products), corn (88%), canola oil (93%, also called rapeseed oil) sugar beets (up to 95%) and Hawaiian papaya (48% Rainbow and SunUp varieties). In 2000, the Grocery Manufacturers Association estimated that 70 percent of the food on grocery shelves contained GE ingredients. Watch out for the most common of these: corn, soy, cottonseed oil, canola oil and sugar beets.

Other Sources of GMOs
- Dairy products from cows injected with rbGH or rbST.
- Food additives, enzymes, flavorings and processing agents, including the sweetener aspartame (NutraSweet®) and rennet used to make hard cheeses.
- Meat, eggs, and dairy products from animals given GM feed.
- Honey and bee pollen that may have GM sources of pollen.

Ingredients That May Be Genetically Modified
Vegetable oil (soy, corn, cottonseed, or canola), sugar (unless organic or cane based) margarines, soy flour, soy protein, soy lecithin, textured vegetable protein, cornmeal, corn syrup, dextrose, maltodextrin, fructose, citric acid, and lactic acid.

A Call to Educators
Why We Should Bring Food to Class

Cynthia Franklin

My interest in taking the topic of GMOs into the classroom started with a call from a reporter from the University of Hawai'i (UH) student newspaper *Ka Leo*. She was working on a story about Monsanto giving money to the College of Tropical Agriculture and Human Resources (CTAHR), and she wanted to know what I thought about this.

Although I teach far afield from CTAHR, in the English department, I did indeed have a strong opinion about Monsanto money. In large part, my response came from my opposition to educators being indebted to corporations (a topic I take up in my research). Taking money from corporations limits – or rather, can influence in troubling ways – the intellectual inquiry that should be at the heart of education and research. In addition, UH is a Land Grant Institute, with responsibilities to the people of Hawai'i, and Monsanto is not just any corporation, but one involved in a number of high profile, class-action lawsuits that involve health and environmental concerns.

When the reporter published her story on CTAHR and Monsanto, she included my commentary. The response to my remarks became the catalyst for my growing investment in education about GMOs. The day after the article appeared, I found an inbox full of extremely uncollegial emails from CTAHR faculty accusing me of being ignorant and full of false anti-corporate biases. The letters to the editor from CTAHR faculty members that followed were more professional in tone, and focused on my lack of understanding about agriculture. After all, their arguments went, I was an English professor – what did I know about GMOs? They implied that I should stick to Shakespeare, and leave the science to CTAHR.

This response, and my sense that I had struck a nerve, got me thinking about just how crucial it is to study GMOs across the curriculum, and in kindergarten through college classrooms. We all eat, and what we eat has enormous implications that go beyond what scientists claim to know about genetic engineering.

Food matters not only because our health directly depends upon what we eat or don't eat, but also because the production of food involves far reaching questions of land, labor and power. To mention but a few examples, whether it be preschool children in Hawai'i who are breathing the herbicides and pesticides sprayed on nearby fields owned by Monsanto; whether it be consumers across the United States eating food that the government and corporations will not label as genetically modified; whether it be farmers in India experiencing economic ruin and taking their own lives in what has been called "GM genocide" because of their dependency on seeds that don't self-reproduce – we all have a stake in what we eat.

The opportunities for education about food in history, political science, sociology, ethnic studies, economics and nutrition classes are as wide ranging as they are urgent, and a wealth of research exists for teachers to use. In any class that teaches writing, critical thinking, research skills, or oratory, food has its place – assignments about food can involve speech and debate, or the writing of poems, position papers, interviews, seminar papers, or letters to newspaper editors and legislators.

What follows is a sampling of ideas to bring food issues into the classroom, so that students and teachers can be more mindful about how and what we eat, and more educated about the many political, economic, environmental, social and cultural ingredients of our food. Scientists can and indeed must study these issues with all the tools at their disposal, but the same goes for the rest of us who share an interest in education and in something as foundational to our existence as food.

Cynthia G. Franklin is professor of English at the University of Hawai'i, where she teaches contemporary ethnic literature and cultural theory. She is also co-editor of the journal Biography, *and the author of* Academic Lives: Memoir, Cultural Theory and the University Today *and* Writing Women's Communities: the Politics and Poetics of Contemporary Multi-Genre Anthologies. *She is currently involved in the UH GMO Education Project and the UH group, Food Sovereignty Hawai'i.*

Teaching Tools
Activities and Curriculum Ideas

Humanities teachers who employ writing as a key learning tool can engage their students with the questions around GE and farming in a number of ways. Following are ideas to encourage critical thinking and analysis of the political, economic and cultural impacts of food production and consumption:

- Narrative writing assignments in general stimulate reflection on the topic of our food systems and how they relate to society, families and individuals.

- Students can seek out and reproduce individual or collective "food stories." This can be done by interviewing family members, chefs, farmers or others about food production, preparation or consumption.

- Letters to the Editor or to legislators about food systems issues are useful exercises for persuasive or argumentative writing.

- Hawai'i's food systems, food security and food sovereignty are rich topics for research papers, and sifting through the variety of sources available – scholarly, oral or media – helps to teach information literacy and critical evaluation of source material.

- History students can analyze the differences and similarities between different agricultural industries in Hawai'i, such as plantation agriculture and today's seed crop industry.

- Debate and/or role-playing exercises help students to explore and assess various sides of the GMO issue. Sample debate topics might include: GMO moratoriums on indigenous food staple plants like taro; corporate funding for public university research; whether or not GMO labeling is just a consumer choice issue, or if government regulation should be involved; whether the planting of GMO test seed crops on designated agricultural lands in Hawai'i should be permitted; etc.

Science teachers can employ a variety of research, testing and analytical methods to make firsthand observations of our local food systems. Taking into consideration grade level and the infrastructural resources available, teachers can apply the issues of farming and GMOs to biology, chemistry and agricultural sciences:

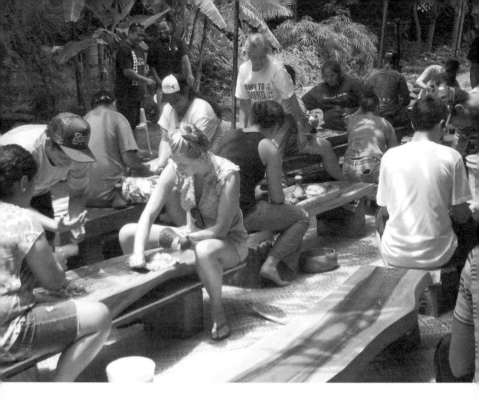

- Students can make qualitative and quantitative comparisons between GE and non-GE foods, both as crops in the field and in their final form as a food product on the market.
- Biology and chemistry students can study the impacts of chemical inputs on different agricultural and ecological systems, including air, water and soil quality.
- Math or economy students can collect and analyze statistics related to the impact of GE agriculture on human health, economies of scale and the environment.
- Economy students can employ the concept of the "triple bottom line" that considers social and environmental health along with economic success to assess different agricultural systems.

There are a variety of curriculum resources that can be used for assigned reading and viewing, including a number of high quality documentary films produced in the last decade on these topics. Please see page 87 for our recommendations.

Take Action!

After reading through this booklet and learning about the realities of GMO food and agriculture in Hawai'i, most people are highly motivated to DO something! You are not alone. Hawai'i SEED and other organizations are working hard on this issue and you can join us.

- *Join Hawai'i SEED's Action Alert List* to keep in touch with our work and stay informed about a range of simple and effective actions that you can take. This might include providing timely testimonies to the legislature, attending public events, and receiving updates on GMO-free foods and the latest activities in Hawai'i. Visit our web site at www. hawaiiseed.org or send us an email at hawaiiseed@hawaiiseed.org.

- If you are a member of a *Community Organization*, have your organization sign on to the statements about a GMO Free Hawai'i that you agree with.[1]

- If you are a *Legislator* or agricultural decision-maker, introduce or support legislation for mandatory labeling of GMO food products and moratoriums on open-air releases of GMO crops until long-term, peer reviewed animal, human health, environmental and agricultural studies can be done to ensure Hawai'i's protection. We can help organize testimony from the outer islands.[2]

- If you are a *Farmer*, refuse to grow GMO crops. Educate other farmers about the problems of GMO farming. Test your papaya trees and chop down your unwanted GMO trees.[3] Let your extension agent and legislators know the reasons why you don't want GMO pollen and seed in your growing environment. Liability for contamination of your crops, loss of markets, high costs of testing, or loss of seed variety lines and ability to save clean seed are among the reasons. Contact Hawai'i SEED for strategies for your industry group to follow to prevent commercial release of a GMO version of your crop such as the coffee and taro industries have done.[4]

- If you are a *Consumer*, shop and eat GMO-free.[5] Refer to the article on page 77 to help you choose GMO-free foods.[6] When you buy papayas, dispose of seeds so they can't grow into GMO trees. Demand labeling of GMO products from your market, manufacturers and governments, so that you can make an informed decision.[7]

- If you are a *Parent*, feed your family GMO-free. These foods have not received adequate safety testing either by the manufacturer or the government regulatory agencies.[8] Schools that feed their children whole foods and have removed GMO foods from the lunch and snack menus have noticed positive change in student behavior.[9] Contact your child's school and ask for these changes. Stay abreast of new research on the health issues surrounding GMO foods.[10]

- If you are a *Citizen*, speak out. Write letters to the editor[11] – this is an easy and direct way that you as an individual can have a big impact on the public discourse that affects policy. Contact your legislators and let them know that this technology has entered the food chain and the ecosystem without sufficient testing and without your permission.[12] Demand mandatory labeling of GM foods. Give volunteer hours or financial support to Hawai'i SEED. Educate yourself and your neighbors about this topic, which is often left out of the mainstream news.

- If you are a *Gardener*, use GMO-free seeds.[13] Ask your county officials if any GMO crops are being grown or tested in your area with crops (especially corn) that could contaminate your family's garden corn crop. Test the papaya trees in your yard and chop down GMO contaminated trees. Save GMO-free seed by bagging a flower of a hermaphrodite tree that you have tested and found GMO-free. The seeds of that fruit will be GMO-free trees, but may get GMO air contamination in their fruits. Let your Cooperative Extension office, Master Gardener program, and County and State lawmakers know that you want to garden in a GMO Free Hawai'i.

- If you are a *Doctor* or healer, educate your patients about the health concerns related to GMO foods and living near GMO crops. When diagnosing, consider effects of a change from GMO-free to GMO ingredients in your patient's diet. Demand that your local public health department track possible allergic and other responses to ingestion or aerosolization of these novel genes. These foods have not gone through the normal regulatory channels of animal testing, human testing and post-market surveys.[14, 15]

Educate Yourself!

Additional Information and Educational Resources

Hawai'i

Hawai'i SEED
www.hawaiiseed.org
Hawai'i SEED is a statewide nonprofit coalition of grassroots groups working to educate the public about the risks posed by genetically engineered organisms and to promote diverse, local, healthy and ecological food and farming.

Earthjustice
www.earthjustice.org/regional/honolulu
Earthjustice is a nonprofit public interest law firm dedicated to protecting the magnificent places, natural resources and wildlife of this earth and to defending the right of all people to a healthy environment.

KAHEA
www.kahea.org
KAHEA advocates for the proper stewardship of our resources and for social responsibility by promoting multi-cultural understanding and environmental justice.

Label It Hawai'i
www.labelithawaii.org
Label It Hawai'i is a grassroots coalition formed to raise awareness and promote labeling legislation in Hawai'i.

Life of the Land
www.lifeofthelandhawaii.org
Life of the Land is a nonprofit environmental and community action public interest group that works to protect the environment in Hawai'i.

Sierra Club
www.hi.sierraclub.org
The Sierra Club is working to restore air and water quality, to protect and restore the land, preserve biological diversity and to conserve our region's resources.

GMO Free Maui
www.gmofreemaui.org
GMO-Free Maui strives to bring people of like interest together in order to see our children and grandchildren grow up in a healthy world.

National

Center for Food Safety
www.centerforfoodsafety.org
CFS engages in legal, scientific and grassroots initiatives to guide national and international policymaking on critical food safety issues.

Californians for GE-Free Agriculture
www.calgefree.org
The Californians for GE-Free Agriculture brings together farmer-based organizations with consumer and environmental groups to halt the introduction of GE crops.

Civil Eats
www.civileats.com
Civil Eats is a daily news source for

critical thought about the American food system. It publishes stories that shift the conversation around sustainable agriculture in an effort to build economically and socially just communities.

Council for Responsible Genetics
www.gene-watch.org
CRG works through the media and concerned citizens to distribute accurate information and represent the public interest on emerging issues in biotechnology.

Environmental Commons
www.environmentalcommons.org
Environmental Commons opposes the uncontrolled expansion of GMOs, and supports communities democratically reaching decisions regarding the adoption and growing of GMO agriculture.

Farmer to Farmer Campaign
www.farmertofarmercampaign.com
The Farmer to Farmer Campaign on Genetic Engineering is a network of farm organizations from throughout the U.S. that seeks to build a farmer driven campaign focused on concerns around agricultural biotechnology.

Farm Aid
www.farmaid.org
Farm Aid helps to keep family farmers on their land to provide fresh, locally grown, healthful food by making grants to farm organizations, churches and service agencies in 44 states.

Food First
www.foodfirst.org
The Institute for Food and Development Policy, also known as Food First, is a "people's think-and-do tank." Its mission is to end the injustices that cause hunger, poverty and environmental degradation throughout the world.

Genetic Engineering Action Network
www.geaction.org
The Genetic Engineering Action Network (GEAN) is a diverse network of grassroots activists, NGOs, farmer and farm advocacy groups, academics and scientists who have come together to work on the myriad of issues surrounding biotechnology.

Indigenous Peoples Council on Biocolonialism
www.ipcb.org
The IPCB is organized to assist indigenous peoples in the protection of their genetic resources, indigenous knowledge, cultural and human rights from the negative effects of biotechnology.

Just Label It
www.justlabelit.org
Hundreds of organizations representing the health care community, consumer advocates, farmers, concerned parents, environmentalists, food and farming organizations, businesses, the faith-based community, and others concerned with protecting the consumer's right to know, have joined together to petition the FDA and demand the mandatory labeling of genetically engineered foods.

National Family Farm Coalition
www.nffc.net
NFFC serves as a national link for grassroots organizations working on family farm issues, including GMOs.

Organic Seed Growers and Trade Association
www.osgata.org

OSGATA develops, protects and promotes the organic seed trade and its growers, and assures that the organic community has access to high quality organic seed, free of contaminants and adapted to the diverse needs of local organic agriculture.

Pesticide Action Network
www.panna.org
PAN North America, or PANNA works to replace the use of hazardous pesticides with ecologically sound and socially just alternatives. As one of five PAN Regional Centers worldwide, it links local and international consumer, labor, health, environment and agriculture groups into an international citizens' action network.

The Institute for Responsible Technology
www.responsibletechnology.org
The Institute for Responsible Technology is a world leader in educating policy makers and the public about genetically modified (GM) foods and crops. It investigates and reports their risks and impact on health, environment, the economy, and agriculture.

The Non GMO Project
www.nongmoproject.org
The Non-GMO Project is a non-profit organization committed to preserving and building sources of non-GMO products, educating consumers, and providing verified non-GMO choices.

The Organic Consumers Association
www.organicconsumers.org
The OCA is a grassroots nonprofit public interest organization which deals with crucial issues of food safety, industrial agriculture, genetic engineering, corporate accountability and environmental sustainability.

The True Food Network
www.truefoodnow.org
The True Food Network is the Center for Food Safety's grassroots action network, where concerned citizens can voice their opinions about critical food safety issues, and advocate for a socially just and sustainable food system.

International

GM Watch
www.gmwatch.org
GM Watch is an independent organization that seeks to counter the enormous corporate political power and propaganda of the biotech industry and its supporters.

GMO Compass
www.gmo-compass.org
GMO Compass is a comprehensive website and database of GMO food-related information that was created within the European Commission's Sixth Framework Programme.

Navdanya
www.navdanya.org
Navdanya is a participatory research initiative founded by world-renowned scientist and environmentalist Dr. Vandana Shiva. Navdanya has created awareness on the hazards of genetic engineering, defended people's knowledge from biopiracy and food rights in the face of globalization.

Books

Your Right to Know: Genetic Engineering and the Secret Changes in Your Food
Andrew Kimbrell (2007)
Genetic Roulette
Jeffrey Smith (2007)
The Omnivore's Dilemma
Michael Pollan (2008)
Uncertain Peril
Claire Cummings (2008)
Making Peace With the Earth: Beyond Land Wars and Food Wars
Dr. Vandana Shiva (2012)
Altered Genes, Twisted Truth
Stephen Druker (2012)

Films

The Future of Food (2004)
The Power of Community – How Cuba Survived Peak Oil (2006)
Islands at Risk (2006)
King Corn (2007)
The World According to Monsanto (2008)
Food, Inc. (2008)
Dirt! The Movie (2009)
Fresh, The Movie (2009)
Vanishing of the Bees (2009)
Living Downstream (2010)
Forks Over Knives (2011)
Bitter Seeds (2012)
Ingredients Hawai'i (2012)
Seeds of Hope (2012)

Photo Credits
by Page Number

5: Kumu Keala Ching. *Photo: Nancy Redfeather.*
7: Hawai'i SEED workshop. *Photo: Marilyn Howe.*
15: Seed corn in Kaua`i. *Photo: Jeri DiPietro.*
19: GMO test site on Kaua`i. *Photo: Jeri DiPietro.*
25: GMO test site on Kaua`i. *Photo: Jeri DiPietro.*
29: Pioneer corn on Kaua`i. *Photo: Jeri DiPietro.*
43: Pesticide sign on Kaua`i. *Photo: Jeri DiPietro.*
45: GMO awareness gathering in Hale'iwa. *Photo: Phoebe Eng.*
47: Organic sunrise papaya on Moloka'i. *Photo: Jeri DiPietro.*
55: GMO fields near the Koloa Sugar Mill on Kaua'i. *Photo: Jeri DiPietro.*
63: Native Hawaiian man circa. 1890. *Photo: public domain.*
65: Walter Ritte at a GMO rally at the Hawai'i State Capitol. *Photo: Jeri DiPietro.*
68: GMO free rally at the Hawai'i State Capitol. *Photo: Jeri DiPietro.*
69: Kūla'ila'i Pūnua Anthony. *Photo: Jonas Maon.*
73: Kauhi Maunakea Forth pounding kalo. *Photo: Jonas Maon.*
75: GMO awareness gathering at Hale'iwa Beach Park. *Photo: Mary Oyama.*
81: Community ku'i kalo day at UH Center for Hawaiian Studies. *Photo: Catherine M. Black*

References by Chapter

What is Genetic Engineering? (Page 8)

1. Statistics on field tests for genetically engineered crops available on the website of "Information Systems for Biotechnology" established as part of the National Biological Impact Assessment Program, a program administered by USDA <www.isb.vt.edu/CFDOCS/fieldtests2.cfm>

2. Hill, J.A., A. Kiessling, R.H. Devlin. 2000. Coho salmon (*Oncorhynchus kisutch*) GE for a growth hormone gene construct exhibit increased rates of muscle hyperplasia and detectable levels of gene expression. Can. J. Fish. Aquat. Sci. 57: 939-50. In "Elements of Precaution: Recommendations for the Regulation of Food Biotechnology in Canada," The Royal Society of Canada, Ottawa, January 2001, p.182, www.rsc. ca/foodbiotechnology/GMreportEN. pdf.
Lindstrom, C.D., T. van Do, I. Hordvik, C. Endresen, S. Elsayed. 1996. Cloning of two distinct cD-NAs encoding parvalbumin, the major allergen of Atlantic salmon salmo salar. Scan. J. Immunol. 44: 335-44.

3. Vanessa E. Prescott, Peter M. Campbell, Andrew Moore, Joerg Mattes, Marc E. Rothenberg, Paul S. Foster, T. J. V. Higgins, and Simon P. Hogan, "Transgenic Expression of Bean- Amylase Inhibitor in Peas Results in Altered Structure and Immunogenicity," Agric. Food Chem., 53 (23), 9023 -9030, 2005.

4. "Australian researchers scrap GM peas after mice fall ill,"AFX News Limited, 17 November 2005

5. "UK Medical Group Urges Moratorium On GM Crops," Reuters 18 May 1999.

6. FDA, "Statement of Policy: Foods Derived from New Plant Varieties," (GMO Policy), Federal Register, Vol. 57, No. 104 (1992), p. 22991.

7. Quoted in Michael Pollan, "Playing God in the Garden," *New York Times Magazine*, October 25, 1998.

8. Benbrook, CM (2003), "Impacts of Genetically Engineered Crops on Pesticide Use in the United States: The First Eight Years," BioTech InfoNet, Technical Paper No 6, Nov 2003, http://wwww. biotech-info. net/technicalpaper6.html.

9. "SEEDless in Seattle," RAFI news release, Rural Advancement Foundation International, 26 November 1999.

10. C. James, "Global Review of Commercialised Transgenic Crops: 1998," ISAAA Briefs No. 8. ISAAA: Ithaca, NY, 1998.

11. Muir, WM, Howard, RD (1999) "Possible ecological risks of GE organism release when transgenes affect mating success: sexual selection and the Trojan gene hypothesis," PNAS 96:13853- 13856. Also see: "Impacts of genetically engineered crops on pesticide use in the U.S. – the first sixteen years," by Charles Benbrook, Environmental Sciences Europe 2012, 24:24. A 2012 study by Charles Benbrook, research professor at Washington State University's Center for Sustaining Agriculture and Natural Resources, found that "GMO technology drove up herbicide use by 527 million pounds, or about 11 percent, between 1996 (when Roundup Ready crops first hit farm fields) and 2011."

12. "Lawsuit Challenges Open-Air Testing of Genetically Engineered 'Biopharm' Crops. USDA Not Adequately Protecting Food Supply," EarthJustice Press Release, November 12, 2003.

Health Effects of Genetically Engineered Food (Page 14)

1. "French experts very disturbed by health effects of Monsanto GM corn," (24/4/2004), http://www. gmwatch.org/archive2.asp?arcid=3308, Translation of Le Monde article "L'expertise confidentielle sur un inquiétant maïs transgénique," Confidential report on a worrying GM corn. Also see Spilling the Beans, June 2005.

2. Mercer, D.K., Scott, K.P., Bruce- Johnson, W.A. Glover, L.A. and Flint, H.J. (1999). Fate of free DNA and transformation of the oral bacterium Streptococcus gordonii DL1 by plasmid DNA in human saliva. Applied and Environmental Microbiology 65, 6-10.

3. Netherwood, et al, "Assessing the survival of transgenic plant DNA in the human gastrointestinal tract," Nature Biotechnology, Vol 22 Number 2 February 2004. http://www.nature.com/nbt/journal/v22/n2/abs/nbt934.html

4. Vanessa E. Prescott, Peter M. Campbell, Andrew Moore, Joerg Mattes, Marc E. Rothenberg, Paul S. Foster, T. J. V. Higgins, and Simon P. Hogan, "Transgenic Expression of Bean- Amylase Inhibitor in Peas Results in Altered Structure and Immunogenicity," Agric. Food Chem., 53 (23), 9023 -9030, 2005. 10.1021/jf050594v S0021-8561(05)00594-7, October 15, 2005:
Mice exposed to alpha-amylase inhibitor of GM-peas showed evidence of an immune response after two weeks, with the response increasing at four weeks. The reaction in mice was evident by inflammation in the lungs and increased serum antibody levels. The research also showed that after eating the GM peas, there was evidence that the pea alpha-am
ylase inhibitor protein primed the mice to react to other food antigens.

5. J. Ordlee, et al, "Identification of a Brazil-Nut Allergen in Transgenic Soybeans," The New England Journal of Medicine, March 14, 1996.

6. G. A. Kleter and A. A. C. M. Peijnenburg, "Screening of transgenic proteins expressed in transgenic food crops for the presence of short amino acid sequences identical to potential, IgE-binding linear epitopes of allergens," BMC Structural Biology, vol. 2, 2002, p. 8-19.

7. Ewen, S.W.B., Pusztai, A., 1999b. "Effects of diets containing genetically modified potatoes express-ing Galanthus nivalis lectin on rat small intestine," Lancet 354, 1353-1354: This study showed that feeding GM potatoes expressing a lectin gene from the snowdrop plant to rats led to major changes in gut structure and function, including thickening of the stomach mucosa and proliferative hyperplastic growth of the rat small intestine leading to crypt enlargement. The genetic modification process ap-peared to be fully responsible for the latter effect and partially responsible for the stomach mucosal thickening, showing the need to test all new GM products for undesirable gastric changes, which at present is normally not done.

8. Joan K. Lemen et. al, Monsanto Company Toxicology Report MSL 18175, "CV-2000-260: 13-Week dietary Subchronic Comparison Study with MON 863 Corn in Rats Preceded by a 1-Week Baseline Food Consumption Determination with PMI Certified Rodent Diet #5 002," 15 December 2002.

9. "Assessment of Additional Scientific Information Concerning StarLink Corn," FIFrA Scientific Advisory Panel to the EPA, SAP Report No. 2001-09, from meeting on July 17/18, 2001.

10. William Freese and David Schubert, "Safety Testing and Regulation of Genetically Engineered Foods," Biotechnology and Genetic Engineering Reviews, Vol. 21, 299-324 November 2004.

11. Mayeno, A.N. and Gleich, G.J. (1994) "Eosinophilia-myalgia syndrome and tryptophan production: a cautionary tale." Tibtech 12, 346- 352.

12. Schubert, D. (2002). "A different perspective on GM food," Nature Biotechnology, Vol. 20, p.969. (From California Certified Organic Farmers Association's report "What is Genetic Engineering?" http://www.ccof.org/ge_mr.php)

Pesticide Use in Crop Biotechnology (Page 17)

1. Schulz, R. 2004. Field studies on exposure, effects, and risk mitigation of aquatic nonpoint-source insecticide pollution: A review. J. Environ. Qual. 33, 419-448.

2. Chang, F.C., Matt F. Simcik, and Paul D. Capel. 2011. Occurrence and fate of the herbicide gly-phosate and its degradate aminomethylphosphonic acid in the atmosphere. Environmental Toxicology and Chemistry. 30(3):548-555.

3. Pimentel, P., Paul Hepperly, James Hanson, David Douds, and Rita Seidel. 2005. Environmental, Energetic, and Economic Comparisons of Organic and Conventional Farming Systems. BioScience. 55(7):573-582..

4. Ibid.

5. GAO. 2001. Agricultural pesticides: Management Improvements Needed to Further Promote Integrated Pest Management. Report to the Chairman, Subcommittee on Research, Nutrition, and General Legislation; Committee on Agriculture, Nutrition, and Forestry, U.S. Senate United States General Accounting Office, GAO-01-815, August 2001. 36 pp.

6. Leffall, LaSalle D., Jr. and Margaret L. Kripke. 2010. Reducing environmental cancer risk: What we can do now, President's Cancer Panel, 2008–2009 Annual Report. National Cancer Institute. 240 pp.

7. Ibid.

8. Pimentel, D., Maria Tort, Linda D'Anna, Anne Krawic, Joshua Berger, Jessica Rossman, Fridah

References   89

Mugo, Nancy Doon, Michael Shriberg, Erica Howard, Susan Lee, and Jonathan Talbot. 1998. Ecology of Increasing Disease: Population growth and environmental degradation. Bioscience. 48:10:817-826.

9. Jasik, C.B. and Robert H. Lustig. 2008. Adolescent Obesity and Puberty: The "Perfect Storm". Ann. N.Y. Acad. Sci. 1135: 265–279; and Holtcamp, W. 2012. Obesogens An Environmental Link to Obesity. Environmental Health Perspectives.120(2)A63-A-68.

10. IOM (Institute of Medicine). 2012. Accelerating Progress in Obesity Prevention: Solving the Weight of the Nation. Washington, DC: The National Academies Press. ISBN 978-0-309-22154-2, 462 pp.

11. Lu, Y., Kongming Wu, Yuying Jiang, Bing Xia, Ping Li, Hongqiang Feng, Kris A. G. Wyckhuys, and Yuyuan Guo. 2010. Mirid Bug Outbreaks in Multiple Crops Correlated with Wide-Scale Adoption of Bt Cotton in China. ScienceExpress. 10.1126/science.1187881. May 13, 2010.

12. Faria, C.A., Felix L. Wackers, Jeremy Pritchard, David A. Barrett, and Ted C. J. Turlings. 2007 High Susceptibility of Bt Maize to Aphids Enhances the Performance of Parasitoids of Lepidopteran Pests. PLoS ONE. 2(7): e600. doi:10.1371/journal.pone.0000600

13. Antoniou, M., M.E.E. Mostafa. H.C. Vyvyan, HC. Jennings, C. Leifert Rubens, O. Nodari, C. Robinson, and J. Fagan. 2011. Roundup and birth defects Is the public being kept in the dark? Earth Open Source. June 2011. 52 pp.

14. Séralini, G.E., Emilie Clair, Robin Mesnage, Steeve Gress, Nicolas Defarge, Manuela Malatesta, Didier Hennequin, Joël Spiroux de Vendômois. 2012. Long term toxicity of a Roundup herbicide and a Roundup-tolerant genetically modified maize. Food and Chemical Toxicology. http://dx.doi. org/10.1016/j.fct.2012.08.005

15. Rodriguez, A.M. and Elizabeth J. Jacobo. 2010. Glyphosate effects on floristic composition and species diversity in the Flooding Pampa grassland (Argentina). Agriculture, Ecosystems and Environment. 138:222–231

16. Brower, L.P., Orley R. Taylor, Ernest H. Williams, Daniel A. Slayback, Raul R. Zubieta and M. Isabel Ramirez. 2012. Decline of monarch butterflies overwintering in Mexico: is the migratory phenomenon at risk? Insect Conservation and Diversity. 5:95-100

17. Valenzuela, H. 2011. Alternatives to the use of Roundup herbicide. Univ. of Hawaii at Manoa, CTAHR, available at: http://dl.dropbox.com/u/33544971/roundup%20alternatives%20HV.pdf.

18. Owen, M.D.K. 2010. New options for weed management in 2010. In: 2010 Herbicide Guide for Iowa Corn and Soybean Production. Iowa State Univ. Revised Agribusiness Education Program, November 2009. WC-94.

19. Alaux, C., Brunet, J.L., Dussaubat, C., Mondet, F., Tchamitchan, S., Cousin, M., Brillard, J., Baldy, A., Belzunces, L.P., and Le Conte, Y. 2010. Interactions between Nosema microspores and a neonicotinoid weaken honeybees (Apis mellifera).Environ Microbiol.12(3):774-82; and Laurino, D., Marco Porporato, Augusto Patetta, and Aulo Manino. 2011. Toxicity of neonicotinoid insecticides to honey bees: laboratory tests Bulletin of Insectology. 64(1):107-113, 2011. ISSN 1721-8861.

20. Valenzuela, H. 2012. Environmental and Health Risks of Synthetic Chemicals used by the Biotechnology Seed Industry in Hawaii. Univ. at Hawaii Manoa, CTAHR. Available at: http://dl.dropbox. com/u/33544971/PesticidesKauaiHV12.pdf

21. Ibid.

22. Ibid.

23. Johal, G.S., and D.M. Huber. 2009. Glyphosate effects on diseases of plants. Europ. J. Agronomy. 31:144-152.

24. Andres, L.A., E. R. Oatman and R. G. Simpson, 1979. Re-examination of pest control practices (Chapter 1). In: D.W. Davis et al (Eds.) Biological Control and Insect Pest Management. University of California, Agricultural Experiment Station. ISBN. 0931876346. Bulletin 1911. 102 pp..

25. GAO. 1992. Sustainable agriculture: Program Management, Accomplishments, and Opportunities. Resources, Community, and Economic Development Division. 8-249128 GAO/RCED-92-233. 50 pp.

26. AliNiazee, M.T., K.S. Hagen and S.C. Hoyt. 1979. Current trends and future outlook (Chapter 12). In: D.W. Davis et al (Eds.) Biological Control and Insect Pest Management. University of California, Agricultural Experiment Station. ISBN. 0931876346. Bulletin 1911. 102 pp.

27. Ibid.

28. McIntyre, B.D., H.R. Herren, J. Wakhungu, and R.T. Watson (eds.) 2009. International assessment of agricultural knowledge, science and technology for development (IAASTD) : Global report. Island Press, Washington D.C. ISBN 978-1-59726-538-6, 606 pp.

29. Owen, M.D.K. 2010. New options for weed management in 2010. In: 2010 Herbicide Guide for Iowa Corn and Soybean Production. Iowa State Univ. Revised Agribusiness Education Program, November 2009. WC-94.

30. Gassmann, A.J., Jennifer L. Petzold-Maxwell, Ryan S. Keweshan, and Mike W. Dunbar. 2011. Field-Evolved Resistance to Bt Maize by Western Corn Rootworm. PLoS ONE. 6(7):e22629. doi:10.1371/journal.pone.0022629; Ives, A.R., Paul R. Glaum, Nicolas L. Ziebarth, And David A. Andow. 2011. The evolution of resistance to two-toxin pyramid transgenic crops. Ecological Applications. 21(2):503–515.

31. Pimentel et al., 2005

32. Panups (Pesticide Action Network North America Updates Service.) 1994. Over 40,000 U.S. Farmers Significantly Reduce Pesticide Use, News Update. August 29, 1994.,

33. Antoniou, M., Claire Robinson and John Fagan. 2012. GMO myths and truths: An evidence-based examination of the claims made for the safety and efficacy of genetically modified crops. Earth Open Source. Available at: http://earthopensource.org/index.php/reports/58.

GMOs in Hawai'i – The Big Picture (Page 25)

1. House Subcommittee on Conservation, Rural Development, and Research Report on the House Hearing on "Review of Agricultural Biotechnology" 6/23/04.

2. http://www.usda.gov/oig/webdocs/50601-08-TE.pdf.

3. Hao, Sean, "Technology Tax Credits Total $108M," Honolulu Advertiser 8/23/05.

4. Kalapa, Lowell, "State Should Reveal Its Tax Credit Beneficiaries," West Hawaii Today 9/18/05.

5. Testimony of the Biotechnology Industry Organization submitted to the Hawai'i Joint Committee on Water, Land, and Agriculture Energy, Environment, and International Affairs 2/10/04 regarding Senate Bills 644,647,649,1037,1847.

Gaining Ground in the Courts (Page 28)

1. Agricultural biotechnology refers to the use of recombinant DNA techniques and related tools of biotechnology to genetically engineer crops used in the production of food, feed, and fiber. The resulting products are referred to interchangeably as "transgenic" or "genetically engineered" (GE) crops and foods.

2. Namely, the Center for Food Safety and its sister organization, the International Center for Technology Assessment, along with the Klamath Siskiyou Wildlands Center, based in Oregon.

3. Specifically, Creeping Bentgrass and Kentucky Bluegrass, two weedy perennial grasses.

4. Namely, the Geertson Seed Farms, Trask Family Seeds, Center for Food Safety, Beyond Pesticides, Cornucopia Institute, Dakota Resource Council, National Family Farm Coalition, Sierra Club, and Western Organization of Resource Councils.

5. To grow sugar beets, seed must first be produced. The seed-producing crop is planted in the fall, and harvested the following summer. The harvested seed is then planted the following spring to produce sugar beets.

6. 7 U.S.C. § 7712(a).

7. 7 U.S.C. § 7701(1).

8. 7 U.S.C. § 7702(10).

9. Id. § 7702(14).

10. 7 C.F.R. § 340.0.

11. Id. § 340.6(d)(3)(i).

12. Almost all of the remaining acreage consists of crops engineered to produce their own pesticide, a toxin derived from the Bacillus thuringiensis (or Bt) bacterium, the DNA of which is inserted into the crops' genetic material. The Environmental Protection Agency (EPA) is also responsible for regulating those crops.

13. Once absorbed by a plant, glyphosate is shunted to the roots, where some is secreted into the surrounding soil, altering the soil biology. Glyphosate kills weeds in part by suppressing plant defenses and fostering infection of roots by prevalent pathogenic soil organisms such as Fusarium fungi.

14. See, e.g., Lands Council v. Powell, 395 F.3d 1019, 1026 (9th Cir. 2005).

15. 50 C.F.R. § 402.14(a).

Public Health and the Regulation of GMOs (Page 41)

1. For the National Academy of Sciences document go to: www.nap. edu/books/0309092094/html/4. html. Go to page 4 and see the graph and legend. From the rest of the text you will see that 3 of the 4 highest risk techniques are GM methods.

Further reading:
Steinbrook R., Financial Conflict of Interest and the FDA's Advisory Committees, NEJM 2005, 353(2);p 116-8.

Wood A.J., Drazen J.M., Greene M.F., A Sad Day for Science at the FDA, NEJM 2005, 353(12); p 1197-9.

GMO Labeling Legislation (Page 45)

1. "How California Could Force the Rest of the US to Label GMO Foods," Mother Jones Magazine, May 31, 2012.

2. "GMO label 'very important'," Honolulu Advertiser, July 12, 2007.

3. "47 Members of Congress Call On FDA To Label Genetically Engineered Foods," Organic View - Volume 1 Number 17.

4. "Fifty-Five Members Of Congress Call On FDA To Require Labeling Of Genetically Engineered Foods," Press Release, Center for Food Safety, March 12, 2012.

5. "Sanders Amendment, What Does it Mean?, "True Foods Network, 6/27/2012: http://truefoodnow. org/2012/06/27/the-sanders-amendment-on-ge-labeling-fails-in-senate-but-what-does-it-mean/

6. "GMO Transparency," Honolulu Weekly, September 26, 2012.

Papaya and Coffee (Page 47)

1. "Big Isle Papaya Crop Tainted," Hawai'i Tribune-Herald, April 7, 2000.

2. National Agriculture Statistics Service www.nass.usda.gov/hi/stats/ stat-28.htm.

3. McNarie, A., "Plenty Papaya Problems," Hawai'i Island Journal, April 1-15, 2003.

4. Elias, P. "New 'gene flow' problems concern crop producers," The Associated Press, September 23, 2004; "Genetic Traits Spread to Non-Engineered Papayas in Hawai'i" September 10, 2004 (Environmental News Service).

5. Identity Preservation Protocol for Non-GMO Papayas. Revised April 16, 2004. Hawai'i DOA, Quality Assurance Division, Commodities Branch.

6. Pollack, A., "Can Biotech Crops Be Good Neighbors?" New York Times September 26, 2004.

Unintended Consequences? (Page 51)

1. See The Fourth National Organic Farmers' Survey: Sustaining Organic Farms in a Changing Organic Marketplace, published in July 2004 www.ofrf.org. Examples of organic farmers impacted by GMOs include: *Laura Krause, an organic farmer in Iowa who grows corn seed for organic growers. In February 2002, she sent her seed to a local lab for routine tests and discovered genetic contamination. She lost her certification, and the price she received for her corn dropped by half – from $3.50 a bushel to $1.75 a bushel. "There's no way for me to go into that field and look for the plants that contain the transgenes and deselect them," said Krause. "There's no way for me to sort them out, because they all look exactly alike. I can't get my business back, because I don't have any way to remove this gene from this [corn] population." (Mark Schapiro, "Sowing Disaster?" The Nation, Oct 28, 2002 www. thenation.com/doc. mhtml?i=200210 28&s=schapiro)

- The Union of Concerned Scientists has estimated that, based on a $0.50/bushel organic price premium and an average organic corn harvest of 120 bushels, contamination could mean a potential lost income of $90 million annually for organic corn growers. This does not take into account the growth of the organic market. ("Union of Concerned Scientists comments to the Environmental Protection Agency on the renewal of Bt-crop registrations," www.biotechinfo.net, 10 September 2001).

- An organic grain processor in Berwick, Ontario refused to purchase organic soybean crops that tested positive for genetic contamination. Farmers were forced to sell the crop for half the cost. ("Genetically altered strains spread by the wind," Alex Roslin, Toronto Star. September 30, 2002.)

- Marc Loiselle, from Vonda, Saskatchewan, describes himself as the "steward of an intergenerational family farm" and has been farming organically for 17 years. He received inquiries from an Asian buyer for organic canola offering C$18/bushel compared to the conventional rate of around C$7/bushel. But he knew it would be impossible to keep his crop free from genetic contamination because of nearby genetically engineered canola fields. In the end he had to plant barley, which meant a loss of C$23,920. Marc is now hoping his losses will be compensated through a class action lawsuit by the Saskatchewan Organic Directorate. (Hugh Warwick and Gundula Meziani "SEEDs of doubt - North American farmers' experiences of GM crops," Soil Association, September 2002)

- Alex Nurnberg, is an organic farmer who was affected by genetic contamination at his 180-acre farm near Ailsa Craig. Tests found 15 to 20 tonnes of his 100-tonne corn harvest had been contaminated by genetically engineered pollen. Tests to uncover the contamination cost Nurnberg $1,000. Insurance is not available to cover his losses. ('Genetically altered strains spread by the wind'. Alex Roslin. Toronto Star. September 30, 2002.)

- The number of farms in Canada growing organic canola was reduced from 200 farms to only one in just two years because of contamination from genetically engineered crops. (Hillary Lindsay, 'Genetically modified crops threaten organic growers,' The Dominion, June 24, 2004 http://dominionpaper. ca/environment/2004/06/24/crop_contr.htm)

2. In 1998, cross-pollination from genetically engineered corn was suspected of contaminating an organic farm in Texas. The contamination was not discovered until the corn had been processed and shipped to Europe as organic tortilla chips under the brand name Apache. By then the company, Terra Prima, had to recall and destroy 87,000 bags. The event cost the small company in excess of $150,000. "FDA holds Oakland hearing to discuss genetic labeling," Oakland Tribune, 14 December. "US Organic Corn Chips Exported to Britain Are Found to Be Contaminated by Genetic Engineered Corn,'" Genetic Food Alert campaign Press Release)

3. The USDA has established no tolerance levels for GMO contamination in organic crops. A Q&A on the USDA website www.ams.usda.gov/nop/Q&A.html makes the following comments about genetic contamination of organic produce: The Preamble to the National Organic Program regulations, Applicability, Clarifications (1) Genetic Drift, states: The presence of a detectable residue of a product of excluded methods [which include GMOs] alone does not necessarily constitute a violation of this regulation. As long as an organic operation has not used excluded methods and takes reasonable steps to avoid contact with the products of excluded methods as detailed in their approved organic system plan, the unintentional presence of the products of excluded methods should not affect the status of an organic product or operation. However, if a certifying agent has reason to suspect that an organic product has come into contact with prohibited substances or been produced using excluded methods, the certifying agent can call for testing, which under certain conditions could result in that product no longer being considered organic."

4. Email communication between Elisha Goodman of Hawai'i SEED and Richard Matthews of USDA NOP, 2004 Referencing section of organic standards 205.202(b)

5. *Ibid.*

From Plantations to GMOs (Page 55)

1. *Ola I Ka Wai: A Legal Primer for Water Use and Management in Hawai'i*, D. Kapua'ala Sproat, a publication of Ka Huli Ao Center for Excellence in Native Hawaiian Law (2010). The legal concepts described in this article are derived from this publication which is also available at http://www.law. hawaii.edu/news/2010/01/25.

2. "Kuleana lands" are often interpreted as those lands which were granted to native Hawaiian tenants pursuant to L. 1850, p. 202 entitled "An Act Confirming Certain Resolutions of the King and Privy Council, Passed on the 21st Day of December, A.D. 1849, Granting to the Common People Allodial

Titles for Their Own Lands and House Lots, and Certain Other Privileges," as originally enacted and amended. *See, for example*, Hawaii Administrative Rules Title 13, Department of Land and Natural Resources Sec. 13.5.2 "Definitions". Also, Kuleana: "right, privilege, concern, responsibility" (from Mary Kawena Puku'i and Samuel H. Elbert, *Hawaiian Dictionary* 179.

3. *Sugar Water: Hawaii's Plantation Ditches*, Carol Wilcox, University of Hawaii Press (1996), pp. 86, 25-26, 33.

4. *Ibid.*, pp. 93-97.

5. Maehara, Eric *Agribusiness Development Corporation: Revisited*. Honolulu, HI: Legislative Reference Bureau (January 2007). See also Kent, Noel *Hawaii: Islands Under the Influence*, Honolulu, HI: University of Hawaii Press (1993).

6. *Ibid.* and See Haw. Rev. Stat. S. 163D.

7. Certain exemptions and powers were given to allow ADC to expedite projects and act more like the private sector. Some of the exemption and powers include: exemption from HRS Chapter 171 (public lands); exemption from the Public Utilities Commission regulations; ability to issue bonds and form subsidiaries. See *ADC Strategic Plan* October 15, 2008. p. 2.

8. Meahara, note 5 and Southichack, Mana, Former *Kekaha Sugar Company Land and Infrastructure: Its Current and Potential Economic Capacity*, Final Report, October 6, 2005.

9. Minutes for the Meeting of the Board of Land and Natural Resources Monday, May 24, 2004. Item D-5. For BLNR decisions setting aside lands and water to ADC, see, for example DLNR Land Division PSF No: 05KD-234 and S-7359. For additional BLNR decisions granting land and water use and management rights to KAA and it members, see for example, Revocable Permit No. S-7252 (2003).

10. *Ibid.*

11. General Lease No. S-3852, Board of Land and Natural Resources.

12. *Restated and Amended Memorandum of Agreement between State of Hawaii Agribusiness Development Corporation and Kekaha Agriculture Association*, dated August 29, 2008. See also Kekaha Agriculture Association Articles of Incorporation dated November 3, 2003.

13. Notice of Amendment to Sole Source Contract, Hawaii State Procurement Office dated February 4, 2009. Sole source reference number 08-013J.

14. *See, for example*, Annual Report, Kekaha Agriculture Association, Department of Commerce and Consumer Affairs; Smaller local leasehold farmers, often within the GMO company formal and informal communities, are invited to farm land and become members of KAA, at the discretion of those GMO companies and the local land manager. Those few local farmers have less influence in KAA, but operationally serve as KAA's public face to the west side community.

15. *See, for example*, Malama Kaua'i, Diversified, Localized, and Sustainable Agriculture on Kaua`i: Assessing Opportunities and Addressing Barriers www.malamakauai.org/docs/AgStudy/MalamaKauai-AgStudy-HighRes.pdf (copy on file).

16. *Agribusiness Development Corporation Grapples with Conflicts over Diverted Water in Kekaha*, Environment Hawaii, Volume 21, Number 11, May 2011. See also License Agreement No. L1-K1101 State of Hawaii ADC as Licensor and PLP as Licensee, dated April 15, 2011.

17. ADC minutes of Kekaha Committee Meeting of September 15, 2010, p. 4.

18. http://www.pacificlightandpower.com/sg_hydro_content/documents/Konohiki_Hydro_Power_FERC_Exemption_Application_Part_2Exhibit_F_G_Appendices.pdf (copy on file)

19. *See, for example*, Leopold Center Fellow, Fred Kirschenmann, in a TEDx presentation: *Soil: From Dirt to Lifeline*, January 21, 2012.

20. See, for example Airaksinen, et al. *Association Between Type 2 Diabetes and Exposure to Persistent Organic Pollutants* (2011). *See also generally* "Pesticides in Our Bodies," http://www.panna.org/issues/persistent-poisons/pesticides-in-our-bodies. *See also* Van Voorhis, *Waimea Residents Sue Pioneer: GMO Seed Company Facing "Substantial" Lawsuit*, The Garden Island, December 13, 2011; *and* various posts on the blog Maluhia Group, such as this post re: pesticides used adjacent to Waimea Canyon Middle School during the 2006-07 school year: http://maluiawcms.blogspot.com/2007/06/pesticide-herbicide-fungicide-101.html.

21. Grubbing: clearing land to remove roots, brush.

22. See, for example Van Voorhis, *Large-Scale Die-off of Sea Urchins Discovered Off Kaumakani*, The

94   *References*

Garden Island, February 12, 2012, and Van Voorhis, *County Takes Legal Action Against Seed Companies: Dow Agro, Pioneer Addressing Unpermitted Grubbing Violations*, The Garden Island, May 3, 2011.

23. Environment Hawaii, Note 16.

24. Stronger state enforcment of water rights generally would include support for commissioned research to understand and perhaps quantify the health care and other longterm social and environmental costs brought about by GMO company and plantation practices.

25. *Environment Hawaii*, Note 16. *See also* Southichack, *An Economic Assessment of Former Kekaha Sugar Company Land and Infrastructure: Its Current and Potential Economic Capability*, Hawaii Department of Agriculture (2005): "…there is more water available than needed…Currently, excess water must be pumped out 24 hours with two pumping stations using hydroelectric power generated within the subject land to keep down the groundwater table to prevent possible root rots." P.15.

26. http://www.pacificlightandpower.com/sg_hydro_content/documents/Konohiki_Hydro_Power_FERC_Exemption_Application_Part_1_Exhibit_A_E.pdf (copy on file).

27. Haw. Const. art XI, S. 7.

28. See Note 2.

29. Appurtenant rights: Rights that attach to parcels of land that were cultivated, usually in the traditional staple kalo, at the time of the Mahele of 1848. Because appurtenant rights attach to the land and not to any individual, they can be exercised by property owners irrespective of race or gender. See Note 1, *Ola I Ka Wai*, p. 10.

30. Haw. Const. art. XI, S. 7. Riparian rights protect the interests of people who live along the banks of rivers and streams to the reasonable use of water from that stream or river on riparian land.

31. Haw. Const. art. XII, S. 7; Haw. Rev. Stat. S. 174C-101(c); Haw. Rev. Stat. S. 174(C)-101(a); and *Waiahole I, 94 Hawai'i at 137-39, 9 P.3d at 449-51 and as affirmed in Na Wai Eha petition to the Commission on Water Resource Management*, State of Hawaii, Case No. CCH-MA06-01 (August 2012).

32. *Waiahole I*, 94 Hawaii at 142, 9 P.3d at 454.

33. *Hawaii Water Code, Article 11*, Sec. 7. This section 7 and section 1 adopts the public trust doctrine as a fundamental principle of constitutional law in Hawai'i. In *Waiahole Combined Contested Case Hearing*, 94 Hawaii 97, 132, 9 P.3d 409, 444 (2000).

34. See Note 28.

35. *Hawaii Water Code Chapter 174(c)-63 and -101; Haw. Rev. Stat. S. 174C-101(c)*.

36. Land division usually extending from the uplands to the sea. Mary Kawena Puku'i & Samuel H. Elbert, Hawaiian Dictionary (1986 ed.).

Take Action! (Page 82)

1. and 2. www.hawaiiseed.org

3. Contact your cooperative extension agent to ask for papaya tree tests. www.ctahr.hawaii.edu/ctahr2001/Counties/HawaiiCounty/faculty. html

4. www.hawaiiseed.org

5. www.seedsofdeception.com

6. www.truefoodnow.org/shoppersguide

7. Contact your legislators at www.hawaii.gov & www.capitol.hawaii.gov

8. www.safe-food.org/index.html

9. www.seedsofdeception.com/GMFree/Campaigns/GM-FreeSchools/ index.cfm; Impact of Fresh, Healthy Foods on Learning and Behavior - 2002. It is available from: Natural Press, P.O. Box 730, Manitowoc, WI 54221-0730. The price of $6 for each tape includes shipping and handling. www.organicconsumers.org/school/ appleton090304.cfm

10. www.seedsofdeception.com

9. www.higean.org/letter-to-editor.htm

11. Contact your legislators at www.hawaii.gov & www.capitol.hawaii.gov

12. www.gmofreehawaii.org

13. GMO-Free SEEDs www.organicconsumers.org/purelink.html

14. www.prast.org Physicians for Social Responsibility

15. hawaiiseed@hawaiiseed.org

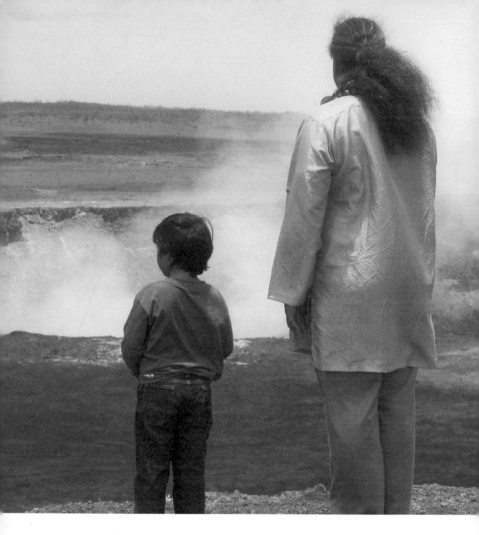

Ho Mai Ka ʻIke

Na Kumu Keala Ching

Ho mai ka ʻike ʻike papalua e	*Grant us the Knowledge to understand both sides*
Ho mai ka ʻiʻini ʻiʻini papalua e	*Grant us the Desire to understand*
Ho mai ka mana mana papalua e	*Grant us Spiritual Insight to understand*
Ho mai, Ho mai, Ho mai Ka papalua e E Ola!	*Grant us the Vision to see both sides* *Let it live!*